Social Indicators Research Series

Volume 92

This series provides a public forum for authored and edited volumes on social indicators research. It is a companion series to the journal Social Indicators Research. The book series deals with problems associated with the quality of life from a broad perspective. It welcomes research on a wide range of substantive areas, including health, crime, housing, education, family life, leisure activities, transportation, mobility, economics, work, religion and environmental issues. The topics represented in this series cover and involve a variety of segmentations, such as social groups, spatial and temporal coordinates, population composition, and life domains. The series presents empirical, philosophical and methodological studies that cover the entire spectrum of society and are devoted to giving evidence through indicators. It considers indicators in their different typologies, and gives special attention to indicators that are able to meet the need of understanding social realities and phenomena that are increasingly more complex, interrelated, interacted and dynamic. In addition, it presents studies aimed at defining new approaches in constructing indicators. An international review board for this series ensures the high quality of the series as a whole.

Available at 25% discount for International Society for Quality-of-Life Studies (ISQOLS).

Sooraj Kumar Maurya

Exploring Justice as a Social Indicator of Life

Philosophical Foundations and Empirical Approaches

Springer

Sooraj Kumar Maurya
Department of Philosophy
Zakir Husain Delhi College (Evening)
University of Delhi
New Delhi, Delhi, India

ISSN 1387-6570 ISSN 2215-0099 (electronic)
Social Indicators Research Series
ISBN 978-3-032-10811-1 ISBN 978-3-032-10812-8 (eBook)
https://doi.org/10.1007/978-3-032-10812-8

This Springer imprint is published by the registered company Springer Nature Switzerland AG
The registered company address is: Gewerbestrasse 11, 6330 Cham, Switzerland

Preface

This book is the outcome of more than a decade of sustained critical engagement with the interrelated concerns of philosophy, justice, and the practical exigencies of governance. As a teacher of social and political philosophy, and as a scholar of affirmative action and moral theory, I have been consistently drawn to a central tension: the persistent gap between the normative ideals of justice and the empirical mechanisms through which societies endeavor to give them effect. The purpose of this book is to address that disjunction: not by reducing justice to quantifiable indicators, but by grounding processes of measurement and institutionalization in a coherent and defensible normative framework.

The animating premise of the study is that justice, though conceptually abstract, must be rendered empirically discernible if it is to meaningfully inform public policy, democratic deliberation, and institutional reform. In an era in which governance is increasingly mediated by metrics and performance indicators, I contend that justice should not be subsumed within technocratic rationalities. Rather, it must function as the normative compass by which the act of measurement itself is directed and evaluated.

In pursuing this aim, the book draws on diverse theoretical traditions: including Rawlsian, feminist, postcolonial, and capabilities-based approaches: while engaging critically with the epistemological assumptions underlying contemporary measurement regimes. It argues for a pluralist yet philosophically rigorous account of justice that can operate across different cultural, political, and institutional contexts. By integrating normative standpoints with empirical applicability, this work aspires to contribute to an emerging interdisciplinary conversation on how societies can responsibly translate the moral demands of justice into tangible, assessable, and action-guiding forms.

New Delhi, India — Sooraj Kumar Maurya

Acknowledgments

Writing a book is a collaborative journey, and this work owes its existence to the guidance, support, and inspiration of many. I am deeply grateful to my colleagues at Ramanujan College and Zakir Husain Delhi College (Evening), University of Delhi, for their intellectual camaraderie, collegiality, and the stimulating conversations we have shared over the years. Your insights during discussions, seminars, and workshops have significantly shaped the trajectory of this work.

I extend my heartfelt thanks to my mentors and teachers, whose wisdom has profoundly influenced my philosophical reflection on affirmative action policy and normative justice. Your guidance has sharpened my understanding and refined my approach to the complex ethical and philosophical questions that underlie this work.

I would like to express my deepest gratitude to my beloved better half, Asha, my Chacha Ji, Ram Prakash Maurya, IRS (Indian Revenue Service), my elder brother, Rajesh Kumar Maurya, and my younger brother, Ravi Maurya, for their unwavering support, patience, and encouragement. Their love and understanding have been a constant source of strength and inspiration throughout this endeavor.

I also wish to recognize the contributions of my dear friends and peers, whose works I have referenced and engaged with in these pages. Your scholarship has provided both foundation and inspiration. In preparing the manuscript, I made selective use of AI-assisted language tools to enhance clarity and flow, while ensuring that all ideas, arguments, and conclusions are entirely my own.

Finally, I dedicate this work to my students: never merely recipients of knowledge but co-inquirers into the deepest questions of justice: and to those whose lives and struggles remind me that the ethical task of justice must remain both philosophical and political.

Contents

1 Justice and Quality of Life: A Philosophical Perspective 1
Introduction 1
Justice: A Philosophical Legacy 3
Quality of Life: Definitions and Debates 5
Intersecting Concepts: Justice as a Social Determinant of Quality of Life 8
Justice Beyond Fairness: Lived Experience and Social Functionality 8
Philosophical Challenges in Measuring Justice 11
Why Justice Must Be Treated as an Indicator 14
The Role of Philosophy in Interdisciplinary Justice Studies 17
Conclusion 19
References 21

2 Theoretical Foundations of Justice 25
Justice and the Question of Foundations 25
Ancient Philosophical Conceptions of Justice 27
The Early Modern Turn: Contract, Reason, and Rights 29
Liberal Egalitarianism and Its Discontents 31
Justice Beyond the Liberal Canon 33
Communitarian Reorientations 33
Feminist Philosophies of Justice 34
Postcolonial and Global Justice Perspectives 35
Justice and Human Flourishing: Virtue, Capabilities, Recognition 36
Justice as a Virtue of Social Institutions and Persons 36
Nussbaum's Capabilities List as an Index of Just Arrangements 37
Axel Honneth on Recognition and Moral Injuries 37
The Interdependence of Agency, Dignity, and Material Conditions 38
Methodological Questions: Ideal Versus Nonideal Theories 39
The Aspirations and Limits of Ideal Theory 39
Nonideal Theory: Realism, Historical Specificity, and Institutional Critique 40

The Demands of Justice in Imperfect, Unjust Societies 40
How Should Philosophy Engage with Empirical Realities? 41
Justice, Structure, and Systemic Power 41
Structural Injustice and the Limits of Individual Blame 42
Ideology and the Reproduction of Unjust Social Orders 42
Intersectionality and Systemic Complexity 43
Moral Responsibility Under Oppressive Structures 43
Cosmopolitan and Transnational Justice 44
Concluding Summary 46
References 48

3 Measuring Quality of Life: Social Indicators Overview 51
Introduction 51
The Necessity of Operationalizing Normative Concepts 51
The Challenge of Complex Human Goods 52
Epistemological Stakes of Quantification 52
Historical Evolution of Social Indicators Research 53
In GDP to GPI: Economic Determinism and the Origins of Counter-Metrics 54
The Post-war Welfare State and the Social Indicators Movement . . . 55
Enlightenment Rationalism and Positivist Influence on Measurement . . . 55
Normative Assumptions in Early Social Science Quantification 56
The Philosophical Foundations of Measurement 57
Ontological Status of Well-Being and Social Goods 57
The Epistemic Tension: Objectivity Versus Subjectivity 58
Conceptual Inquiry: "Well-being," "Welfare," "Utility," "Capability," "Functioning," "Life Satisfaction" 59
The Problem of Value Commensurability: Pluralism and Measurement 59
Key Frameworks for Measuring Quality of Life 60
The Utilitarian-Subjectivist Tradition 61
The Capabilities Approach 62
The Human Development Index (HDI) and Beyond 63
OECD Better Life Index, Gross National Happiness (Bhutan), and the SDGs 63
Critical Perspectives on Quantification and Objectivity 64
Foucault: Measurement as a Technology of Biopower and Governmentality 65
Bourdieu: Symbolic Violence and the Epistemic Power of Indicators . . . 66
Cartwright and Morgan: Models the Slimness of Models and Limits of Quantification 66
Coloniality of Knowledge: Who Measures, and For Whom? 67
Justice, Distribution, and the Ethics of Indicators 68
Indicators as Distributive and Recognitional Tools 68
The Ethical Dimensions of Aggregation 69

Procedural Justice and Epistemic Inclusion 69
Indicators as Instruments of Public Reasoning.................. 70
Challenges in Integrating Justice into Quality-of-Life Measurement... 71
Justice as Indicator or Meta-Norm? 71
Disaggregating Justice-Oriented Metrics: Inputs, Outputs, Outcomes, and Capabilities 72
The Risk of Moral Reductionism 72
Hybrid Approaches: Combining Quantitative Rigor with Qualitative Depth 73
Toward a Philosophical Framework for Ethical Social Indicators 73
Transparency, Reflexivity, Contestability, and Pluralism 74
The Need for Epistemic Pluralism 74
Indicators as Tools of Critique, Not Just Assessment............. 75
Toward Moral Progress, Not Administrative Simplification........ 75
Concluding Summary.. 76
Between Abstraction and Operationalization 77
Quantification as a Moral and Epistemic Practice 77
Looking Forward: Justice as a Social Measure of Quality of Life ... 78
References.. 79

4 Justice as a Social Indicator 83
Introduction.. 83
Historical and Philosophical Context 85
Justice in Classical Philosophy: Seeking Order and Harmony...... 85
Modern Theories: From Morality to Measurability 85
Moral Justice Versus Statistical/Social Justice 86
Influence on Quality-of-Life Paradigms and Social Indicators 87
What Makes a Good Social Indicator?.......................... 87
Objectivity: The Mirage of Neutrality 88
Measurability: The Limits of Quantification 88
Policy Relevance: Technocracy Versus Transformative Potential.... 89
Cultural Sensitivity: Navigating Universality and Pluralism 89
Conceptualizing Justice as a Social Indicator..................... 90
The Multidimensional Nature of Justice: Beyond Redistribution ... 91
A Conceptual Framework for Justice Indicators................. 92
Normative Challenges: Justice to Whose, of Whom, and on What Grounds? 93
Operationalizing Justice: Methodological Considerations........... 94
Quantitative Versus Qualitative: False Binaries and Hybrid Approaches 94
Measuring Perceptions: Surveys as Moral Thermometers 95
Institutional Metrics: Mapping Structural Capacities............. 95
The Cross-Cultural Challenge: Universal Aspirations or Moral Imperialism?... 96
The Nordic Countries Procedural Justice and the Welfare State Context 97

India: Affirmative Action, Caste Equity, and Legal Justice Context ... 98
South Africa: Postapartheid Justice and the Politics of Repair Context ... 99
Comparative Reflections: Patterns and Pitfalls ... 100
Critiques and Limitations of Justice as a Social Indicator ... 101
The Subjectivity and Variability of Justice Perceptions ... 101
Risk of Politicization in Justice Metrics ... 101
Universalism Versus Cultural Relativism: Whose Justice? ... 102
Ethical Critique: Should Everything Be Quantified? ... 102
Future Pathways and Recommendations ... 103
Toward Institutional Integration: Justice in Global Frameworks ... 103
Interdisciplinary Collaboration: Philosophers, Data Scientists, and Policy-Makers ... 104
Participatory Justice Metrics and the Democratic Imperative ... 105
Areas for Future Research and Development ... 105
Concluding Summary ... 106
References ... 107

5 Empirical Studies Linking Justice and Well-Being ... 111
Introduction: The Normative-Empirical Nexus ... 111
From Philosophical Ideal to Lived Condition ... 112
Well-Being as an Ethically Loaded Construct ... 112
The Potential and Dangers of Combining Normative Justice and Empirical Evidence ... 113
Justice and Subjective Well-Being: Correlational and Causal Claims ... 114
Experimental and Longitudinal Studies on Procedural Justice ... 115
Hedonic Versus Eudaimonic Well-Being: Philosophical Challenges ... 116
Distributive Justice and Economic Inequality ... 117
Empirical Links Between Inequality and Social Pathologies ... 117
Critiques: Causal Ambiguity and Cultural Mediation ... 118
Cross-National Comparisons: Nordic Versus Anglo-American Models ... 119
Philosophical Stakes: Efficiency or Justice? ... 119
Recognition, Social Identity, and Psychological Well-Being ... 120
Recognition, Misrecognition, and the Self: Honneth's Normative Framework ... 121
Empirical Evidence of Recognition Theory: Stigma, Exclusion, and Identity Harm ... 121
Marginalization and Mental Health: Race, Gender, and Caste ... 122
Psychological Correlates of Just Treatment: Dignity, Respect, and Agency ... 122
Moral Injury, Collective Trauma, and Post-Conflict Injustice ... 123
Institutional Trust, Justice, and Democratic Participation ... 124
Procedural Justice and Civic Trust: Empirical Evidence ... 124
Legal Empowerment and Access to Justice ... 125

Democratic Legitimacy and Fairness in Allocation: Experimental Insights 125
Normative Interpretation: Compliance or Moral Community? 126
Global South Perspectives: Justice and Well-Being in Development Contexts 126
Critiques of Western Metrics: Epistemological and Ethical Limits 127
Participatory Action Research and Local Conceptions of Justice. . . . 127
Gender Equity and Justice as Empowerment 128
The Ethical Imperative of Epistemic Justice. . . . 129
Capabilities, Functionings, and Multidimensional Well-Being 130
Operationalizing Capabilities: HDI, IHDI, and OPHI Indices 130
Household and Individual-Level Capability Data. . . . 130
Disparities in Capability Distribution: Gender, Caste, and Region 131
Conceptual Tensions: Aggregation, Commensurability, and Reification 132
Justice Metrics and Policy Impact Evaluation 133
Evaluating Redistributive, Affirmative, and Empowerment Policies . . . 133
Conditional Cash Transfers (CCTs) 134
Policy Feedback Loops: When Indicators Reshape Governance 134
Philosophical Critique: Are Outcomes a Proxy for Justification? . . . 135
Methodological Reflections: Limits of Quantification in Capturing Justice 136
Internal Critique: Sampling Bias, Cultural Translation, and Metric Reification 136
Mixed Methods as an Epistemic Imperative. . . . 137
Value Pluralism and the Problem of Incommensurability 138
Normative Guidance Without Instrumentalization 138
Concluding Summary 139
Toward a Normatively Embedded Empiricism. . . . 140
Empiricism as Ethical Praxis: A Philosophical Reframing. . . . 141
Looking Ahead: From Philosophy to Policy Practice. . . . 141
References. . . . 142

6 Justice in Health, Education, and Environmental Policy 145
Introduction. . . . 145
Public Goods, Political Sites: Health, Education, and the Environment 145
Why Sectoral Justice Matters: Beyond Aggregative Measures 146
The Philosophical Challenge: Reconciling Justice Paradigms 147
Justice in Health: Ethics, Access, and Agency 148
Distributive Justice and the Right to Health 148
Empirical Evidence and Policy Practices 149
Normative and Methodological Challenges 150
Justice in Education: Equality, Recognition, and Human Development. . . 151
Philosophical Theories of Educational Justice 151

Empirical Dimensions and Global Indicators 152
Methodological and Ethical Reflections 153
Justice and the Environment: Intergenerational and Global Ethics 154
Environmental Justice as Distributive and Procedural Claim 154
Empirical Studies and Justice Metrics 155
Normative Tensions 157
Cross-Sectoral Intersectionality: Compound Injustices and Policy Synergies 158
Gendered and Racialized Experiences Across Sectors 159
Integrated Justice Frameworks: From Siloed Policies to Multidimensional Interventions 160
Synergistic Policy Action: Contingent Transfers, Eco-Pedagogy, and Green Social Contracts 160
Institutional Ethics and Democratic Accountability 161
Democratic Participation in Policy Design: Whose Voices Count? 162
Indicators and Public Reasoning in Sectoral Governance 162
Transparency, Accountability, and Moral Legitimacy 163
Concluding Summary 164
References 166

7 Philosophical Reflections on Justice Metrics 169
Introduction: Why Metrics Need Philosophy 169
Indicators and the Technocratic Turn in Justice Discourse 169
The Philosophical Task: Interrogating Metrics as Moral Constructs ... 170
Justice Metrics as Ethically Charged Instruments 170
The Ontology of Justice and the Problem of Quantification 172
Is Justice a Measurable Entity or a Regulative Ideal? 172
The Ontological Gap Between Moral Value and Empirical Proxy ... 173
Toward an Ontologically Responsible Philosophy of Measurement ... 174
Indicators as Epistemic Authority 175
Objectivity, Bias, and Epistemic Exclusion 176
Toward Epistemic Democracy in Justice Metrics 177
The Normative Architecture of Measurement 178
The Ethical Fabric of Metrics: What Does and Does Not Get Counted 178
Cartwright and Hardie on "Thick" Concepts in Policy Models 179
Composite Indicators and the Illusion of Neutrality 179
Indicators as Moral Gatekeepers 180
The Politics of Visibility: What Metrics Reveal and Conceal 181
Foucault: Metrics, Biopolitics, and Governmentality 181
Bourdieu: Symbolic Violence and the Imposition of Norms 182
Moral Erasure Through Aggregation 183
Justice as a Meta-Norm: Can It Be an Indicator? 184
The Problem of Operationalization and the Risk of Reification 184
Toward Hybrid Metrics and Informational Pluralism 185

Pluralism, Contestability, and Democratic Design 186
Democratic Legitimacy and the Co-Construction of Metrics 186
Participatory Approaches: Deliberation, Narrative, Experience 187
Reflexivity and Ethical Responsiveness 188
Justice Beyond Measurement: Alternative Ethico-Political Paradigms . . . 188
The Limits of Quantification: Questioning the Epistemic Empire . . . 188
Justice Without Metrics: Ethics of Care, Recognition, and Testimony . . . 189
Critique of Indicator-Centric Governance 189
Justice as Praxis: Responsiveness, Repair, and Historical Consciousness 190
Radical Traditions: Ethics Without Quantification 190
Philosophical Guidelines for Ethical Justice Metrics 191
Conclusion 192
References 193

8 Toward a Just Society: Indicators for the Future 195
Introduction: The Future of Justice as a Measurable Ideal 195
Indicators as Generative, Not Merely Reflective, Tools 196
Normative Criteria for Future Justice Indicators 197
Anticipatory Governance and the Ethics of Forecasting 198
Global Justice and Post-Western Epistemologies 200
Integrative Justice Metrics: Transversality Across Sectors 202
Institutional Ethics and Democratic Accountability 205
Integrative Justice Metrics: Transversality Across Sectors 207
Participatory Indicator Frameworks: Institutionalizing Democratic Epistemologies 210
The Role of Technology and AI in Justice Metrics 212
Philosophical Reorientation: Beyond Perfectionism, Toward a Critical Utopianism 214
Concluding Summary 216
The Moral Architecture of Future Indicators 217
From Descriptive Statistics to Normative Imagination 218
From Quantification to Ethical Orientation 218
References 219

Chapter 1
Justice and Quality of Life: A Philosophical Perspective

Introduction

Historically, ideas about justice have mainly come from moral and political philosophy, whereas quality of life (QoL) is mainly studied in economics, sociology, and public health. Despite the differences, the increase in difficult global issues like inequality, problems with the environment, and overall discrimination makes it necessary for countries to work together. The chapter works to shift the conversation by clarifying that justice is not only a value but also a key element in shaping quality of life. To achieve this, we must think deeply about social issues because many standard social indicators do not capture important ethical issues. In philosophy, justice refers to the ideas that guide how resources and opportunities are distributed among people in a community. Many thinkers in ancient Greece considered justice to be necessary for living a good life and this standpoint was often described through harmony and structural concerns for justice (Aristotle, 2009; Plato, 1991). Currently, theories of justice focus on the rights of individuals, the obligations people have in contracts, and supporting what is best for society as a whole. For instance, Rawls (1971) argued that to achieve justice, we should regard fairness and assure that disadvantages in life help those who are most at risk. However, Amartya Sen and Martha Nussbaum have pointed out that justice is found in the actual capabilities someone has to live the way they wish (Nussbaum, 2011; Sen, 1999).

Alternatively, quality of life (QoL) is generally understood with the help of empirical approaches. In the middle of the twentieth century, quality of life (QoL) was assessed by looking at income, literacy rates, life expectancy, and the availability of public services. By introducing the Human Development Index (HDI) in 1990, the United Nations Development Programme (UNDP) shifted the focus from simple economic data to a wider consideration of human development. For instance, The Better Life Index created by the Organisation for Economic Co-operation and Development (OECD), and the Social Progress Index developed

S. K. Maurya, *Exploring Justice as a Social Indicator of Life*, Social Indicators Research Series 92, https://doi.org/10.1007/978-3-032-10812-8_1

by the Social Progress Imperative (a US-based, non-profit organization) now consider self-perceived well-being, the environment, and civic engagement. Yet, these indicators usually do not consider justice as an important aspect, rather they are inclined to state or describe what is right, rather than assessing or measuring it.

This distinction between these two fields also greatly impacts how policies are put into place. It is common to use quality of life (QoL) indicators for decision-making in development and social programs, yet their bones of normative content are not very apparent. For this reason, philosophical reflection or understanding is essential and cannot be left out of real research. It can guide us in determining the relevant indicators, the importance of those measures, and how they relate to fundamental values like dignity, freedom, and equality. Following Sen's (1999) viewpoint, development includes the expansion of substantive freedoms, instead of superficial gains in income or comfort, and achieving this demands justice across different levels of society. Despite being at the heart of many social theories, justice is still not well developed as a social indicator. Methodologically, justice is challenging to quantify because it has many sides, is tied to values, and depends on culture. It is also said that, philosophically, social scientists view justice as an idea that is hard to measure with statistics or use in causal studies. Alternatively, according to Ziegler and Schwanen (2011), it is possible to carefully apply justice standards to areas such as transport, housing, health care and education. It allows us to grasp in detail how social organizations either help or harm quality of life for several groups of people.

The underrepresentation of justice in empirical studies also represents the wider cultural thinking about it. In the current age of leadership, being efficient and measurable becomes more important than being fair and inclusive. These issues can result in policies reproducing or making worse injustices that were overlooked since time immemorial. It is possible that while a city is very competitive and modern in its digital setup, it might also face problems with racial segregation, limited services in certain districts, or unequal city planning. As long as justice-sensitive indicators are absent from measurements, the purpose of quality of life (QoL) assessment cannot be fully achieved.

To bridge this gap, it is necessary to design a dual approach that combines the principles of philosophy with the analytical methods used in the humanities and social sciences. It is important to regard Justice as responsible for our conduct and as something that helps shape the world such as health, education, environmental support, political involvement, and similar factors. An inquiry of philosophy can fine-tune the concepts and values found in quality of life (QoL) indicators, whereas research provides evidence and verifies their meaning in various contexts. Essentially, justice must be translated, now, from being an idea in books or speeches to concrete action. It needs to be seen as a primary aspect in assessing and understanding quality of life. When we do this, we improve how social indicators are defined and ensure they represent the life situations, goals, and rights of people across society, especially those who have historically been disadvantaged. Therefore, this chapter leads into a more in-depth look at how justice can be an essential factor in creating a society that is just and flourishing.

Justice: A Philosophical Legacy

Both as an idea and a significant part of social structure, justice has played an important role in the development of human thinking and society. It has actual influence over existing social, political and cultural institutions, and is an ideal driver of day-to-day activities. It follows the transformation of justice within philosophical traditions, from simply being a moral virtue to become the standard for assessing social and institutional arrangements.

In classical Greek thought, justice was closely tied to cosmological views that highlighted order, balance, and the rational principles underlying all things. Plato was among the earliest philosophers to describe justice as important for both individual and social well-being. In *The Republic,* Plato envisions a just society as one where each class performs its designated function in harmony with the whole: rulers govern through wisdom, auxiliaries uphold courage, and producers provide for material needs with temperance (Plato, 1991). In this approach, justice means that each class of society has its role, with reason leading, spirit assisting, and appetite following, much like in our inner harmony. For him, justice is both part of society and a metaphysical aim : a representation of the Good that is essential for the well-being of the community, and gives purpose to all thing.

Aristotle, following the teachings of Plato, gave justice a more practical and everyday focus. In *Nicomachean Ethics*, Aristotle distinguishes between general justice (aligned with lawful conduct and virtue) and particular justice, which he further divides into distributive and corrective justice (Aristotle, 2009). In distributive justice, goods, honors, and resources are given out fairly, taking into account what each person deserves or requires. Corrective justice, by contrast, focuses on rectifying injustices in transactions, whether voluntary (e.g., contracts) or involuntary (e.g., theft). Aristotle's emphasis on proportional equality laid the groundwork for later discussions about fairness and equity, while his acknowledgment of social roles and civic responsibility prefigured communitarian theories in modern discourse.

The change from classical to modern philosophy led to a shift in how justice was understood, from its focus on virtue and benefiting the community to respecting individual rights and agreements among people. This transformation corresponds with the rise of the modern state, liberalism, and secular legal institutions(Ruggeri et al., 2020). Following the chaos of civil war and political upheaval, Thomas Hobbes argued that justice should be defined in a way that guarantees stability and authority. In *Leviathan,* Hobbes argues that in the state of nature, where individuals are guided by self-preservation and rational fear, life is "solitary, poor, nasty, brutish, and short" (Hobbes, 1996). It is only through the formation of a social contract and the appearance of a government that justice can exist in Hobbes' view. It relies on agreements and not on absolute moral rules, all of which are protected by a powerful nation. Consequently, justice comes down to obeying the law in a society ruled by an absolute government. John Locke, who came shortly after, puts forward a more positive and rights-centered position. In *Two Treatises of Government*, J. Locke conceptualizes justice as respect for natural rights: life, liberty, and property, that preexist political society (Locke, 1988). The state, created by agreement, is meant to look after these rights. According to Locke, justice ensures that laws are applied fairly to defend freedom and private property, leading to liberal democracy and a constitution.

Jean-Jacques Rousseau critiques both Hobbesian authoritarianism and Lockean liberalism by introducing the concept of the general will in *The Social Contract* (Rousseau, 1973). According to Rousseau, justice arises when people come together to legislate for the good of everyone, leaving aside their own interests. Unlike Locke, who thinks private property supports active societies, Rousseau believes it leads to inequality and divides people. Justice, according to his ideas, means citizens should participate actively in forming the moral and political rules that apply to them. This idea that justice should reflect the views of all people continues to shape modern talks about equal rights and community acceptance.

Contemporary Theories: Fairness, Capabilities, and Recognition

Over the twentieth and twenty-first centuries, discussions about justice in philosophy have addressed subjects such as the fair distribution of resources, developing capabilities, concerns about identity and recognition. Among the most influential voices is John Rawls, whose *A Theory of Justice* (Rawls, 1971) revitalized political philosophy by offering a robust framework for assessing justice in liberal societies. Rawls proposes that principles of justice should be chosen behind a "veil of ignorance" in an "original position," where individuals are unaware of their own social status, abilities, or personal goals. Under these conditions, rational agents would select two principles: (1) equal basic liberties for all, and (2) social and economic inequalities arranged to benefit the least advantaged (the "difference principle"). In Rawls' system, fairness means ensuring basic liberty and also equal treatment when it comes to sharing benefits and burdens.

In his work with Rawls' principles, Amartya Sen raised concerns about the emphasis on perfect theory and building institutions. In *Development as Freedom* (Sen, 1999), Sen argues that justice must be evaluated not solely by rules or resources, but by the actual capabilities people have to pursue valuable lives. The "capability" approach of Sen focuses more on what people actually can do and become, rather than looking at resources or rights they own. According to Sen, "justice" means making sure people have more genuine freedoms by tackling obstacles like poverty, illiteracy, and discrimination based on gender. The capability approach has strongly affected development economics and policy-making, especially through the beginning of the Human Development Index.

Nancy Fraser merges the concepts of distribution and recognition within the discourse. In *Justice Interruptus* (Fraser, 1997), Fraser critiques theories that focus solely on material redistribution or cultural identity, arguing instead for a three-dimensional approach: (1) redistribution to correct economic injustices, (2) recognition to address status hierarchies, and (3) representation to ensure political voice. It is especially valuable for recognizing the relationship between justice and gender, race, disability, and worldwide inequality. Fraser's framework also responds to postmodern critiques of universalism by grounding justice in both structural reform and participatory parity (Böhm et al., 2022).

In all these phases of history, the idea of justice is understood as something that exists within structures, customs, and daily decisions made by governments. The duty to justice is about creating situations where people and communities can maintain their dignity and autonomy. The change from traditional to modern approaches in theories of justice reflects the rising complexity in society and calls for multiple ways of examining problems. Law-making, schooling, businesses, and government bodies are not only tasked with administering justice; but also play a role in defining it. In other words, justice happens when institutions are set up and followed carefully and when they are answerable for their decisions. This insight has led scholars like Iris Marion Young (1990) to emphasize the "structural" nature of injustice, whereby systemic processes, rather than isolated acts, perpetuate inequality. Consequently, the concept of justice needs to connect with the process of moral judgment and the re-looking at the nature of institutions. To include, justice in empirical studies, is used as a sign or indicator of how pleasant life is. However, the researchers must approach it from both descriptive and prescriptive perspectives. It should reliably produce moral judgments and sense while being able to understand the real-life situations that shape our moral decisions. Through initiatives for healthcare, equal access to education, or access to clean air and water, the concept of justice pushes us to reflect on and question contemporary views on human life.

Quality of Life: Definitions and Debates

The concept of quality of life (QoL) occupies a central place in contemporary debates across philosophy, social science, economics, and public policy. Essentially, QoL attempts to capture the degree to which individuals and communities experience life as fulfilling, meaningful, and supportive of their aspirations. However, despite its frequent invocation in global development discourse, the term remains complex, contested, and multidimensional. This is the reason; it becomes essential to outline the evolution of quality of life (QoL) from economic-based models such as Gross Domestic Product (GDP) to more holistic frameworks like the Human Development Index (HDI), contrasts subjective and objective indicators of well-being, and explores the philosophical foundations of human flourishing. It ultimately argues that justice is not a peripheral concern but a constitutive and essentially substantive element underpinning all meaningful and desirable interpretations of quality of life (QoL).

From GDP to HDI: Traditional Measures and Their Limitations

In the past, the main measure of national progress or improvement was the state of the economy, with GDP being the top priority. It shows the total monetary value of goods and services produced in a nation within a specific period. While this measure provides empirical insight into economic activity, it fails to account for inequality, environmental degradation, unpaid labor, or the distribution of well-being across populations (Stiglitz et al., 2009). So, a considerable number of experts and critics argue that GDP fails to capture important aspects of how people live, such as quality of life, and inequality. Due to the constraints mentioned, economists developed new frameworks in the latter part of the twentieth century. The most influential among these is the Human Development Index (HDI), developed by the United Nations Development Programme (UNDP) in 1990. HDI combines three dimensions: life expectancy, educational attainment, and per capita income, offering a more comprehensive picture of human well-being (UNDP, 1990). At the same time, HDI has come under criticism, just like other indexes. It may obscure intra-national inequalities, lack of sensitivity to cultural differences in value-system, and insufficiently integrate dimensions such as environmental sustainability, political freedom, and gender equity. More recent attempts to refine quality of life (QoL) metrics include the Multidimensional Poverty Index (MPI), the OECD's Better Life Index, and the Social Progress Index (SPI), developed by the Social Progress Imperative (a US-based, non-profit organization). They add new dimensions to consider, like safety, housing, work–life balance, ways to be involved in the community and the state of the environment. However, these tools most often think justice, particularly distributive and procedural justice; as implied or secondary, rather than the fundamentally desirable starting point. If there is no single authority for justice, these indices may present a distorted view of how well people are doing, especially in stratified societies.

Subjective Versus Objective Indicators of Well-Being

One important question in quality of life (QoL) research is what factors should be valued more, subjective or objective indicators. Income, health, work situation, housing, and education level are all considered objective measures because they are observable and factual. They aim to create a similar and convenient system in all parts of the world. In contrast, subjective measures focus on individual experiences, perceptions, and evaluations, such as life satisfaction, happiness, and a sense of purpose (Diener et al., 2018). Even though objective measures are dependable and comparable, they cannot always reflect what individuals really go through. Two people with the same income and health situation could still have very different feelings of well-being because of their personal, cultural, or mental differences. Subjective indicators, on the other hand, are context-sensitive and capable of illuminating aspects of quality of life (QoL) that quantitative metrics often overlook, such as emotional well-being, social cohesion, or spiritual fulfillment (Veenhoven, 2000).

However, these steps can also be affected by people adjusting their responses or giving answers that please the interviewer. It is important to consider that good living conditions and how people feel are essential for overall well-being. As Alkire (2005) observes, a purely subjective approach risks downplaying structural inequalities, while a purely objective one may ignore personal agency and preferences. Therefore, to fully assess quality of life (QoL), we should combine these two types of indicators, considering the norms about what makes life worth living.

Philosophical Foundations: Eudaimonia, Dignity, and Autonomy

The philosophical underpinnings of quality of life (QoL) predate modern indicators and can be traced to classical conceptions of human flourishing. The Aristotelian notion of eudaimonia, often translated as "flourishing" or "living well," remains foundational. For Aristotle, a good life is not merely one of pleasure or wealth but one of virtuous activity in accordance with reason (Aristotle, 2009). Eudaimonia entails the actualization of human potential within a community and emphasizes the importance of ethical development, education, and civic participation.

In modern philosophy, the Kantian emphasis on dignity and autonomy provides a complementary foundation. Immanuel Kant (1997 argued that human beings possess intrinsic value or worth and should always be treated as ends in themselves, never merely as means. This ethical framework supports quality of life (QoL) paradigms that center human agency, moral worth, and the capacity for self-determination. The capability approach, developed by Amartya Sen and further elaborated by Martha Nussbaum, integrates these philosophical reflections by focusing on what people are actually able to do and be; their substantive freedoms to live lives they have reason to value and this reflects the true measure of human well-being and capability (Nussbaum, 2011; Sen, 1999). This shift from utility or resource-based approaches to capability and functioning marks a critical development in quality of life (QoL) theory. It foregrounds the normative question: What should people be able to achieve? Rather than prescribing a singular vision of the good life, the capability approach allows for pluralism while insisting on basic thresholds of justice and dignity. As such, it provides a framework that bridges philosophical theory and policy practice.

Justice as the Ethical Core of Quality of Life

Even with so many indicator and metrics used, many quality of life (QoL) frameworks are not strongly rooted in values. They spend more effort on measurement than on questioning what and why something needs to be measured. This is where the concept of justice becomes indispensable. The ethical understanding of QoL centers around justice rather than simply being an additional concern. Even if a society shows significant empirical growth in areas like, GDP, in certain areas, it may still lack high quality of life if economic exclusion or inequality is widespread.

Quality of Life (QoL) indicators are best understood by using justice as the guiding perspective. For example, access to health or school services depends on making sure the resources are used equally and meet local cultural needs. Similarly, political participation and freedom of expression are not just metrics of democratic performance but indicators of procedural justice and recognition (Fraser, 1997). As Young (1990) has shown, structural injustices, such as marginalization, powerlessness, and cultural imperialism, can persist beneath the surface of seemingly prosperous societies. Understanding quality of life (QoL) without considering justice can lead to simply another political notion. As a result, justice ought to be considered in QoL frameworks both as a goal and as something essential to achieving QoL. To do this, we need indicators that include fairness in distribution, fairness in decision-making, and respect for differences among people. It calls for active engagement of marginalized individuals in because everyone's experiences matter. This method of studying uses philosophy to confirm that well-being, necessary for human growth, must be achieved justly.

Intersecting Concepts: Justice as a Social Determinant of Quality of Life

Today, justice is more often seen as an active force that helps shape important aspects of human well-being and development rather than just an abstract normative goal. Traditionally, justice has been conceptualized in terms of fairness, whether in the form of equitable distribution (Rawls, 1971), recognition of cultural identity (Fraser, 1997), or expansion of human capabilities (Sen, 1999). However, justice must also be understood as functionality in lived experience, where individuals' day-to-day realities are shaped by the just or unjust organization of society's institutions, policies, and norms. This functionalist view of justice reveals it as both a determinant and a measurable aspect of quality of life (QoL), thereby necessitating its inclusion in any holistic evaluation of societal well-being.

Justice Beyond Fairness: Lived Experience and Social Functionality

It is important to see how justice or its absence actually makes people feel to fully realize its role in well-being. Fairness is still considered as a desirable idea, but it should also consider access, agency, dignity, and taking part in decisions. As Young (1990) argues, a just society does not merely treat individuals equally in a formal sense; it must also dismantle systemic barriers that impede some groups from fully participating in social, economic, and political life. Being just in our experiences goes beyond having legal protection or formal rights. It involves equitable access to essential goods, such as education, health care, environmental safety, and civic inclusion that directly influence individuals' ability to lead meaningful lives. If people do not have the equal or same access to goods (services) or if they cannot find them, it leads to diminished quality of life (QoL), regardless of other indicators of wealth. Therefore, being just matters both in terms of fairness and in terms of social order.

Structural Justice as a Foundation for Quality of Life

It is structural justice that focuses on the ways and methods that social and political institutions decide how primary and secondary goods or things are distributed among individuals. This standpoint moves beyond individual interactions to consider how systems operate over time to either reproduce or mitigate inequality (Anderson, 2010). Structural justice demands scrutiny of how policies, social norms, and institutional practices affect people's ability to develop and exercise capabilities. Just structures in society make sure that everyone can use important resources for a decent quality of life. For example, Fraser (2008) emphasizes the interdependence between redistribution (economic justice), recognition (cultural justice), and representation (political justice) as integral to justice. They combine to create the structure by which people are able to reach well-being. When structural justice is not guaranteed, people may experience greater and greater obstacles. A child growing up in poverty in a place with environmental problems, little access to schools and poor medical facilities is a good example. In spite of legal rights, the child struggles to achieve a good quality of life because of systemic barriers. Sen's (1999) capability approach emphasizes this idea by focusing on what individuals are actually able to do and to be, highlighting the need to dismantle structural obstacles to attain the well-being.

Empirical Domains of Justice and Quality of Life (QoL)

To concretize the role of justice as a social determinant of quality of life (QoL), it is useful to explore specific domains, such as education, health care, environmental justice, and political inclusion, where its influence is most visible and measurable.

Education

Education helps individuals become independent and improves the progress of a society. Despite the benefits of education, access to education remains restricted to those with strong economic, gender, racial, and social backgrounds. A just educational system not only provides equal opportunities for enrollment but also ensures inclusive pedagogy, equitable distribution of resources, and recognition of diverse learning needs (Nussbaum, 2006). Inequality in schools may appear as insufficient fundind, imbalanced lessons or policies that block people from advancing. Literacy levels, enrollment statistics, and educational gains can all be seen as mechanisms for judging justice in education. UNESCO (2021) reports that children from low-income households, rural communities, and marginalized ethnic groups are disproportionately excluded from quality education, resulting in lifelong disadvantages in health, income, and civic participation.

Health

Health care is another important area where justice plays a direct role in quality of life (QoL). When people have difficulty getting health care due to their income, where they live, gender, or disability, it leads to them having less chance of living a healthy life. The World Health Organization (WHO, 2008) identifies health inequity as one of the most persistent forms of injustice globally. Having access to health services alone is not considered desirable; other factors to consider include the ability to pay, sensitivity to cultural backgrounds, and the right to be included in health choices. Empirical research has shown that social determinants such as housing, education, employment, and nutrition significantly impact health outcomes, highlighting the need for integrative, justice-oriented health policies (Marmot, 2010).

Environment

Environmental justice means sharing out how clean the air is, the quality of water, access to green areas, and protection from pollution. Structural injustices often result in marginalized communities being exposed to higher levels of pollution, climate vulnerability, and resource scarcity (Bullard, 2000). In the context of quality of life (QoL), environmental quality is very much essential to human life and well-being. If the environment is not conducive to the well-being of human beings, the quality of health, mental state, and ability to earn a living can deteriorate, mainly for people relying on nature. Moreover, environmental degradation intersects with intergenerational justice, as it compromises the quality of life of future generations (Gardiner, 2011).

Political Inclusion

People have a right and a need to take part in civic and political life. A person has political inclusion if they can vote, be selected for important government posts, and share their opinions. Exclusion from political processes often correlates with social and economic marginalization, perpetuating cycles of disempowerment (Young, 2000). Indicators such as voter turnout, representation of marginalized groups in legislatures, and freedom indices (e.g., civil liberties, press freedom) provide empirical insights into the state of political justice. Promoting justice in administration helps create trust among people and helps authorities respond well to a wide variety of community issues.

Justice Ensures Both Fair Processes and Equitable Outcomes

To be just, we need both fair methods for making decisions and fair results from those decisions. A society can have transparent legal processes but still fail to deliver justice if those processes consistently yield outcomes that favor the privileged and marginalize the disadvantaged (Rawls, 1971). On the other hand, reaching equality though unclear or pressured tactics could mean that the result is not trusted or can end up being short-lived. To illustrate, some social welfare measures may make people better off materially but not include them in making or carrying out the policies, which can weaken their independence and self-respect. Similarly, anti-poverty programs that fail to consider cultural appropriateness may reinforce dependency or stigma rather than fostering empowerment (Sen, 2009). In other words, when judging justice, we need to study how resources are spread, the decisions made, who joins in such decisions, and what happens to social groups as a result. This idea of justice is very similar to the way we make quality of life (QoL) assessments multifaceted and aware of cultural issues.

Philosophical Challenges in Measuring Justice

For a long time, justice has played an essential role as an important concept in social and political philosophy. It's importance is seen in how it is part of normative and prescriptive reasoning, political thinking, and legal systems across the globe. Still, once justice is studied using quantitative or statistical methods, it leads to many philosophical challenges, and moot questions. Can justice be measured without diminishing its moral richness? Can abstract ideals be translated into tangible indicators? These questions bring up issues around how we know things, disagreements between norms and facts, and the possible flaws in treating justice as a countable quantity. The main concern of this section is to discuss the challenges, and moot questions associated with measuring justice, including considerations of value-laden perspectives, and normative ethics.

Is Justice Measurable? The Epistemological Tension

It is a subject of great discourse and disagreement when normativity is linked to individual action; as justice is constitutive of normative ethics, all of which are rested on standards, values, and virtues that direct moral understanding of individuals, and debated moral beliefs. Justice, unlike inflation or GDP, does not have an automatically recognizable way to be measured. Instead, its understanding is filtered through competing normative traditions, such as, utilitarianism, deontology, capabilities theories, all of which establish different conceptions of the just and justness or righteousness (Fraser, 1997; Rawls, 1971; Sen, 2009). This moral conflict occurs because justice is not something that can be measured from a sole normative lens. According to Nagel (1991), the concept of justice involves questions of "what ought to be," not merely "what is." Thus, it becomes a category of 'Ought' that is context-dependent and can vary for each person, situation, and period, depending on culture, society, and politics. Therefore, the measuring justice begins with a deep understanding what justice really entails. Whose conception of justice is used? Can measurement accommodate plural and sometimes conflicting perspectives? Moreover, when justice is understood as connected to interpersonal relationships or systems, instead of being viewed as a quality of one individual, the conceptualization of justice becomes significantly more complex, and intriguing. Structural injustices, such as systemic racism, gender inequality, or environmental injustice, operate through complex institutional mechanisms that are often hidden, diffuse, and not easily reducible to numerical proxies (Young, 1990). Therefore, relying on statistics in this area may oversimplify the issue of justice (With reference to certain numerical indicators), resulting in a false impression of certainty, while moral uncertainty remains.

The Problem of Normativity Versus Objectivity

One of the main conflicts in quantifying justice is formed by the differences between normativity and objectivity. The concept of justice is related to what is seen as fair, right, and just or in other words, what is "normative." Objectivity, by contrast, is typically understood as value-neutral, empirical, and replicable, a standard demanded by most quantitative research paradigms (Flyvbjerg, 2001). Turning justice, a normative concept, into something measurable produces several issues that require careful consideration. The process often involves the selection of specific dimensions (e.g., income, health, legal access), weighting of those dimensions, and aggregation into composite indices. Estimating what is right, how generous a learning organization should be, and what is tolerable in its missions all require making these kinds of judgments. As an illustration, the Gini coefficient is often used to assess income equity, which is commonly regarded as an indicator of how equal justice is. However, this measure says little about how income is earned, whether it reflects merit or exploitation, or whether inequalities are justified in broader ethical terms (Wilkinson & Pickett, 2009). It is also true that gauging legal access by legal aid clinic numbers alone may not tell you if people from poor groups feel included and secure in the justice system. As Sen (2009) contends, objectivity in evaluating justice must be "positional," sensitive to social context and human experience, rather than absolute or purely procedural. Therefore, avoiding prejudice does not diminish the important normative and ethical dimensions of justice; rather, it is necessary to upholding fairness and equity within a just system.

Can Justice Be Disaggregated into Indicators Without Losing Its Ethical Essence?

Philosophers also debate whether it is possible to dissect justice into merely empirical or numerical components, such as income fairness, equal access to education and government services and yet still retain its complete meaning. Attempting to disaggregate justice into separate parts could hide its true normative meaning and may cause it to lose its cohesion and unity with the holistic understanding of well-being. Justice indicators usually capture the interconnectedness of various essentials that form a just society, further complicating its empirical measurement. For example, the World Bank might use indicators such as the percentage of women in the workforce or how many are enrolled in school to judge gender justice. However, such proxies can be misleading. If more women participate, the ongoing challenges of gender-based violence, unequal childcare duties, or workplace biases might still exist but remain hidden. The complexity of justice, particularly in intersectional contexts, defies neat compartmentalization (Crenshaw, 1991). Also, if we use reductionism, justice can be seen as just following a list of rules instead of being driven by its principles. As Merry (2011) notes, indicators tend to produce "governance through numbers," where quantitative tools shape not just assessment but also action, often reinforcing dominant paradigms and obscuring alternative voices. However, if we view disaggregation through a critical and normative lens, it can still play a positive role. Indicators that are freely described, state their principles openly, and draw on qualitative information are able to expose injustice and lead to progress. For example, the use of disaggregated data in the Sustainable Development Goals (SDGs) has highlighted disparities across gender, income, and geography, prompting targeted policy responses (UN, 2015). Nevertheless, they should be understood as limited guides, not as complete substitutes for normative judgment.

The Value-Ladenness of Metrics: A Double-Edged Sword

All indicators should be understood in the terms of value and virtue bearers; reflecting the underlying normative principles they aim to measure. They involve selecting what is to be measured, setting important thresholds, and using data in the best way possible. Being value-laden is not a failure of social metrics; it is simply a key aspect. As Douglas (2009) and Sen (1999) argue, even the most ostensibly "neutral" indicators embed normative assumptions, about human needs, priorities, and social goals. Acknowledging the value-ladenness of metrics demands philosophical vigilance. It means identifying whose morals are embedded, whose needs are prioritized, and who ultimately benefits from the system. Metrics aren't only used for explaining things; explaining things; they also serve to measure, evaluate, and guide decisions based on quantifiable data; they also influence policy decisions, control the use of available resources, and give legitimacy to choices. Injustice can occur when there are no metrics as well as when metrics are used in the wrong way. If we use statistics that ignore ethics or hide who is more powerful, we may inadvertently support the injustices we seek to overcome. For instance, a metric that measures poverty strictly in terms of income may miss dimensions of deprivation such as social exclusion, insecurity, or lack of voice (Alkire & Santos, 2010). For this reason, it is important to handle the presence of values in research, not by excluding them, but by including more people, working across fields and checking for ethics. Indicators should be used ethically, rather than just as numbers on a page.

Why Justice Must Be Treated as an Indicator

The idea of justice, usually viewed as a guiding framework, is now widely considered as an essential tool to examine and assess human development and policies. While justice has long been a central moral value for philosophers, current challenges on a global scale like inequality and damage to the environment suggest that we need to involve justice not only in decisions about what is right but also in our ways of measuring different contexts and traditions. It argues that development plans should consider justice as a measure that can be counted and also judged. It explains that justice must be seen as central to human well-being and to how policies are created and carried out. If justice is not measured, the signs of injustice are hard to find in government. Thus, having justice defined and measured helps advance social development that is ethical, fair, and proven by evidence.

Justice as Both Qualitative and Quantifiable

Both philosophy and empirical evidence must be combined to assess justice as an indicator. Philosophically, justice is a complex and value-laden ideal encompassing fairness, equality, recognition, and accountability (Rawls, 1971; Sen, 2009). Still, as a matter of observation and assessment, justice should be expressed in terms that can be applied and compared in different societies. This translation requires taking several moral aspects into account instead of flattening the ethical issues; as a result, it helps assess principles in real-life situations. Sen (1999) sets forth a critical starting point through his capability approach, which frames justice in terms of what individuals are substantively free to do and be. In contrast to resource-centered principles, the capability approach considers factors such as reading ability, health, rights in political matters, and safety in nature, which show both the qualitative meaning and measurable aspects of justice issues. Nussbaum (2011) furthers this by proposing a list of central human capabilities that should be secured for every person as a matter of justice, offering a foundation for structured yet ethically resonant measurement. Importantly, viewing justice as both an ideal and a process supports the idea that justice is more than just achieving a result. Qualitative approaches, using ethnographic research, participatory action, or looking at cases, can highlight how injustice is experienced firsthand, but quantitative methods, by using indices, measuring access, and tracking legal action, reveal larger patterns in injustice. Both impact and injustice are necessary for fully incorporating justice into evaluations, ensuring that both measurable outcomes and unfairness are considered in the assessment process.

Justice and Its Impact on Human Development Indices

Human Development Indices (HDIs) and related measurement tools have evolved considerably over the past few decades, transitioning from narrow economic metrics to multidimensional evaluations. However, justice is either neglected or treated as a minor point in the majority of these indices. Not considering justice is significant because it directly and indirectly shapes the four main areas measured by these indices: health, education, income, and political freedom. For instance, education outcomes are deeply influenced by systemic biases, such as racial segregation, linguistic discrimination, or economic exclusion (UNESCO, 2021). Health metrics may conceal disparities rooted in environmental racism or gender-based health care access (Marmot, 2010). Political indicators may reflect formal structures of democracy while failing to capture whether marginalized communities experience meaningful participation (Michalos & Land, 2018).

They demonstrate that justice helps or prevents the development of people and communities. Furthermore, if we don't have justice-sensitive indicators, our assessments could show one-sided and unilateral results. Even if a nation scores considerably high in human development, there may be injustices such as caste divisions or the punishment of people who criticize the government. For instance, the gap between descriptive criteria, such as economic growth or development and normative criteria, such as progress, which shows positive transformation in terms of values and virtues; was evident during the Green Revolution in Punjab (India) and Haryana (India), While these Indian states saw significant economic growth during that time, this growth also led to a decrease in the sex ratio. This is the reason; when descriptive indicators of development or growth are considered without integrating normative aspects concerning individuals, they fail to present a true picture of progress. Consequently, public policies often exacerbate existing gaps rather than address them, as unnoticed injustices remain unrecognized and are not brought to the attention of decision-makers.

Invisibility in Indicators = Invisibility in Governance

This is essentially true in public policy, where what is measured can be more effectively managed in terms of it's efficacy. How governments allocate funds, set priorities, and assess their achievements largely depends on the performance of the metrics used. Without justice being an integral part of these public policies and strategies; the challenges faced by marginalized communities often remain unnoticed in statistics (descriptive indicators) and are frequently overlooked by legislators, failing to receive the attention they ought to deserve. This absence or invisibility has real-world consequences when it comes to the formulation of public policy, as these policies often overlook essential elements and aspects that contribute to the challenges inhibiting the holistic well-being of marginalized communities. For example, consider urban housing policy, without disaggregated indicators that track tenure security, forced evictions, or access to basic services by ethnicity, class, or migration status, policies may benefit the urban elite while displacing informal settlers (Michalos & Land, 2018). Similarly, if indicators of economic development fail to capture labor exploitation or unpaid care work, the burden borne by women and low-income workers is systematically erased from public consciousness and policy discourse (Kabeer, 2005).

Furthermore, the lack of justice indicators hampers accountability. If justice benchmarks are excluded from development plans, governments and institutions cannot be held responsible for their wrongdoings. By incorporating justice in the indicator framework, democracy becomes more transparent and good governance is accomplished. There are various recent models that explain the ways justice can be used as an evaluation tool. Sen's capability approach is perhaps the most well-known, having influenced the HDI and numerous adaptations such as the Multidimensional Poverty Index (Alkire & Santos, 2010). They consider that income is not enough to show how much people lack and that justice involves examining their abilities based on their situations (Maurya, 2025). The Social Inclusion Index is also a helpful model used to gauge what hinders people from participating in society, the economy, and politics. The European Social Inclusion Indicators, for instance, monitor disparities in access to education, employment, housing, and health care, with attention to ethnic minorities, immigrants, and people with disabilities (Atkinson et al., 2002). These indicators are built on morality and carefully carried out with research, proving that both aspects can exist together.

In Latin America, the Social Progress Index (SPI) includes measures of opportunity, access to information, personal rights, and tolerance, aiming to complement traditional economic metrics with justice-sensitive categories (Porter et al., 2014). The OECD's Better Life Index encourages citizens by giving them the option to assign importance to matters like civil engagement and achieving a healthy work–life balance, allowing justice to enter their personal understandings of well-being. These studies show that it is possible to measure and share justice more broadly. The inclusion of justice improves equality and makes policy frameworks suitable for each context. It directs the growth conversation from creating the best results to shaping human values. It is important to focus on justice as a key measurement, rather than an accessory value. The failure to consider race in major development theories blinds authorities to structural problems and negatively affects our view of development. Considering justice as both qualitative and quantifiable helps build an honest, inclusive, and ethical method of measuring quality of life. By merging serious philosophy with established evidence, policy, and practice can support justice in their decisions.

The Role of Philosophy in Interdisciplinary Justice Studies

Philosophy (ethics) has a specific and important role in interdisciplinary studies related to justice. Since contemporary scholarship promotes bringing together theories and research, philosophy gives the intellectual foundation needed for strong ethics-based projects. The understanding of justice advanced by ethics helps both in conceptual thinking and in genuinely guiding ideas in economics, sociology, public policy, and law. It discusses the major importance of philosophy in working with multiple disciplines and explores how combining philosophy with scientific research can ensure knowledge is practical and aligns with social values. One vital contribution made by philosophy is breaking down difficult concepts (Maurya, 2024). Justice is a contested concept, what Gallie (1956) called an "essentially contested concept,"meaning that its definition is always subject to interpretation, debate, and ideological framing. Philosophy helps unpack these complexities by interrogating underlying assumptions, drawing distinctions among types of justice (e.g., distributive, procedural, restorative), and evaluating the internal coherence of competing theories (Nozick, 1974; Rawls, 1971; Sen, 2009). If philosophical clarity is missing, it's easy for interdisciplinary studies to arrive at concepts of justice that are flawed or based on questionable ethics. For instance, treating justice merely as income redistribution might neglect questions of recognition, participation, or institutional trust (Fraser, 1997). With the help of philosophy, we can make sure that justice is recognized as involving more than one dimension in any situation. Its role is to keep research across disciplines clear, well-structured, and mindful of ethical issues.

Normative Benchmarks and Ethical Critique

Philosophy establishes the methods and principles that gives the very idea of standards to evaluate the concepts and theoretical frameworks available to run the major and minor social and political institutions. Although these descriptive disciplines, such as economics and political science might uncover patterns, correlations, and possible causes, they generally avoid stating whether the used theories and principles are desirable or not with reference to the given socio-economic conditions. This normative gap can only be filled by the normative disciplines, such as ethics and logic, they are equipped with the kinds of methods and principles, and have potential to critically evaluate the desirability of used empirical theories and principles with reference to the given socio-economic contexts. Hence, philosophy and its disciplines, such as ethics provides standards to guide us in deciding which social conditions should be encouraged and which should be transformed for greater and holistic well-being. For instance, the Rawlsian principle of "justice as fairness," which includes the equal liberty principle and the difference principle, offers a normative standards for evaluating whether institutional inequalities are morally permissible (Rawls, 1971). Likewise, Sen's (2009) capabilities approach provides an alternative normative foundation that assesses justice in terms of substantive freedoms rather than material resources. Not only do these frameworks analyze unfairness, but they also help in designing institutions that are just. Philosophy also involves examining the indicators that demonstrate social success or failure. It leads us to consider what we are measuring, as well as why and for whom (Land & Michalos, 2018).

It reveals the ethical implications of choosing one metric over another and urges transparency about value-laden assumptions embedded in empirical research (Douglas, 2009). As a result, philosophy controls justice studies, preventing them from concentrating too much on techniques and losing sight of ethics.

Normative philosophy provides fundamental norms and guidelines for evaluation, but it does not exist in a vacuum; it is shaped by cultural, and historical contexts that influence how justice and fairness are understood. When it is connected to areas like economics, sociology, law, and public policy, its true benefits are very much palpable. Through normative philosophy, ideas are clarified in the sense that gives a value inquiry, exploring the normative implications and desirability of those ideas; it helps us assess what is morally right or wrong, what should be prioritized, and what ought to be pursued; on the other hand, social sciences focus on empirical tools to understand, analyze, and apply these ideas in real-world settings, enabling us to create tangible change based on those values. When doing welfare reflection in economics, it is often assumed that utilitarianism is the basis and it tries to maximize the total utility of society. Philosophical critique has shown the limitations of such approaches, particularly their failure to account for distribution, autonomy, or fairness (Sen, 1985). This field has greatly improved by including philosophy-based ethical approaches such as capabilities and justice in its economic models. In sociology, structural theories of injustice, such as those concerning class, race, or gender, gain normative depth when informed by philosophical discussions on equality, recognition, and social obligation (Anderson, 2010; Young, 1990). Using philosophy to look at rights, duties, and procedural justice can help improvc both interpreting the constitution and making new laws. In many cases, public policy is guided by practicality and expense, often ignoring morals. This issue can be addressed by incorporating normative reasoning, which provides a moral framework to ensure that policies are not only effective but also morally consistence and sound. According to Sandel (2009), policy decisions inherently embody moral choices, whether acknowledged or not. With philosophy, the unseen norms of government can be brought to light, promoting greater transparency and accountability in decision-making.

Methodological Synergy: Conceptual Analysis Meets Empirical Tools

Both philosophical and empirical research affect each other and cannot exist without the other. Using concept analysis, researchers can be more focused when asking questions, choosing indicators that suit them and analyzing their data following ethical guidelines. In addition, empirical research helps to prove, improve, or doubt philosophical claims by connecting them to actual experiences and their results.

Mixed-method approaches illustrate this synergy effectively. To illustrate, talking to individuals using justice theories from philosophers can help us understand how individuals see things as fair or unfair. It is possible to use quantitative research to evaluate if democratic engagement or equal access to education improves the well-being outcomes of societies. Participatory action research can integrate community values with philosophical deliberation, co-producing knowledge that is both epistemically robust and democratically legitimate (Flyvbjerg, 2001). Furthermore, interdisciplinary justice studies benefit from what Nussbaum (2006) calls "philosophical humanism," an approach that respects the subjectivity and dignity of research participants, resisting the tendency to reduce them to data points. Justice studies are made deeply humanistic thanks to philosophy's focus on respect, responsibility, and reflexivity. In justice studies, philosophy is meaningful and plays a real role. By offering well-defined ideas, clear guidelines, and ethical analysis, it helps us engage with justice thoroughly and in a significant way. When philosophy teams up with the empirical sciences, it helps us see social reality as a place where justice is needed and not only debated. The combination of normative reflection, and the use of empirical data provides the most promising way for justice research to develop in the twenty-first century.

Conclusion

In conclusion, this chapter has laid a foundational understanding of the intricate connection between justice and quality of life (QoL). It has pointed out that justice should not only exist in philosophical ideas but should be seen as something that influences and can be measured in our day-to-day lives. This theme has been studied from many normative viewpoints, starting with the ancient Greeks (Plato and Aristotle) and more recently by John Rawls, Amartya Sen, and Nancy Fraser. This chapter makes it clear that justice has transitioned from a moral quality to a key part of society, but has always played an important role in enabling individuals and groups to live well and meaningfully (Maurya, 2022).

At the forefront of this theme is the idea that justice is both real and necessary in social systems, rather than just an abstract concept. The way resources, opportunities, and rights are shared in society often affects schooling, health services, government involvement, and environmental policies. With this in mind, the chapter points out that true understanding of justice is more than just theories and needs to be measured in daily experiences worldwide. In this chapter, we see how justice changed from an idea of harmony in ancient times to modern attitudes that stress human rights and the good of the community. Plato saw justice as social harmony with everyone in their own role, which later thinkers drew on (Maurya, 2021). Aristotle used Plato's theories as a base and came up with ideas about distributive and corrective justice to promote fairness of resources and fix injustice. In today's world, writers like Thomas Hobbes, John Locke, and Jean-Jacques Rousseau have shaped justice theories using ideas of social contracts, individual rights, and the general will. There has been a movement away from focusing mainly on virtues toward protecting rights and ensuring fairness in how benefits and burdens are shared in society.

Contemporary theories of justice, with John Rawls, Amartya Sen, and Nancy Fraser as key examples, have added more detail to the debate by talking about justice related to people's abilities, social acceptance, and how goods are divided. Rawls' theory of fairness, which concentrates on helping the groups with the least, and Sen's approach, which aims to allow people to live a life that matters to them, have changed the view of justice as it relates to living standards. On the other hand, Fraser points out that distribution, recognition, and representation are all related, underlining the importance of social justice in economics as well as in cultural and political life. These new views have increased the importance of justice, as it helps shape the quality of life for people, mainly where societies are working toward equity, inclusion, and environmental protection.

While we need these philosophical ideas to understand justice, the chapter has pointed out that measuring justice with data is not easy. Justice is a key idea based on moral standards and understanding it often requires detailed ethical thought. The chapter discussed the conflicts that arise when justice is regarded as normative but also needs to be understood as objective. Since justice covers several moral viewpoints like utilitarianism, deontology, and the capabilities approach, it cannot be accurately counted or measured easily. Nonetheless, as outlined in the chapter, it is possible to operationalize justice by studying its impact in areas where its presence and outcomes can be noticed and measured. To examine justice in education, one might look at the number of people who can get quality schooling, how resources are distributed, and how inclusive the educational policies are. In a similar way, the justice of health care can be checked by exploring if health care is accessible to all and if it is delivered equally among various social groups. Ensuring environmental justice is about giving every community the same safety and clean living conditions, while political inclusion takes into account how much individuals and groups are able to take part in politics. They demonstrate that justice plays a role in improving life quality, proving that it should be prioritized in theories and public policies (Maurya, 2020).

It also made it clear that indicators such as GDP, which are usually associated with quality of life (QoL), do not take into account ethically desirable aspects of human life. The shift from economic-based models of development to more holistic frameworks like the Human Development Index (HDI) and the Social Progress Index (SPI) is a step toward acknowledging the multifaceted nature of quality of life. They tend to not consider justice a core part of their systems. If frameworks do not look at justice-sensitive aspects such as fairness and how decisions are made, they risk hiding inequalities and continuing unjust practices. If there are gaps in measuring policy results, the privileged usually get the benefits while leaving marginalized groups behind. For this reason, this chapter supports replacing the traditional view of justice as a moral principle with one that measures justice as a key indicator used to create better policies and practices for everyone. It states that both unfairness in processes and inequality in outcomes should be looked at through the quality of life (QoL) metrics. As a result, justice reveals differences in society, affects laws and government actions, and supports an inclusive and enduring future. Having justice-sensitive indicators will assist in making certain that social development addresses both progress and the welfare of those who have historically lacked opportunities.

References

Alkire, S. (2005). Subjective quantitative studies of human agency. *Social Indicators Research, 74*(1), 217–260. https://doi.org/10.1007/s11205-005-6525-0

Alkire, S., & Santos, M. E. (2010). *Acute multidimensional poverty: A new index for developing countries*. Oxford Poverty & Human Development Initiative Working Paper Series (38). https://doi.org/10.2139/ssrn.1815243.

Anderson, E. (2010). *The imperative of integration*. Princeton University Press.

Aristotle. (2009). *Nicomachean ethics* (W. D. Ross, Trans.). Oxford University Press.

Atkinson, A. B., Cantillon, B., Marlier, E., & Nolan, B. (2002). *Social indicators: The EU and social inclusion*. Oxford University Press.

Böhm, S., Carrington, M., Cornelius, N., Djelic, M. L., Jones, C., & Mermet, L. (2022). Ethics at the Centre of global and local challenges: Thoughts on the future of business ethics. *Journal of Business Ethics, 180*, 835–861. https://doi.org/10.1007/s10551-022-05239-2

Bullard, R. D. (2000). *Dumping in Dixie: Race, class, and environmental quality* (3rd ed.). Westview Press.

Crenshaw, K. (1991). Mapping the margins: Intersectionality, identity politics, and violence against women of color. *Stanford Law Review, 43*(6), 1241–1299. https://doi.org/10.2307/1229039

Diener, E., Oishi, S., & Tay, L. (2018). Advances in subjective Well-being research. *Nature Human Behaviour, 2*(4), 253–260. https://doi.org/10.1038/s41562-018-0307-6

Douglas, H. (2009). *Science, policy, and the value-free ideal*. University of Pittsburgh Press.

Flyvbjerg, B. (2001). *Making social science matter: Why social inquiry fails and how it can succeed again*. Cambridge University Press.

Fraser, N. (1997). *Justice interruptus: Critical reflections on the "postsocialist" condition*. Routledge.

Fraser, N. (2008). *Scales of justice: Reimagining political space in a globalizing world*. Polity.

Gallie, W. B. (1956). Essentially contested concepts. *Proceedings of the Aristotelian Society, 56*, 167–198. https://doi.org/10.1093/aristotelian/56.1.167

Gardiner, S. M. (2011). *A perfect moral storm: The ethical tragedy of climate change*. Oxford University Press.

Hobbes, T. (1996). In R. Tuck (Ed.), *Leviathan*. Cambridge University Press. (Original work published 1651).

Kabeer, N. (2005). Gender equality and women's empowerment: A critical analysis of the third millennium development goal. *Gender and Development, 13*(1), 13–24. https://doi.org/10.1080/13552070512331332273

Kant, I. (1997). *Groundwork of the metaphysics of morals* (M. Gregor, Trans.). Cambridge University Press. (Original work published 1785).

Land, K. C., & Michalos, A. C. (2018). Fifty years after the social indicators movement: Has the promise been fulfilled? *Social Indicators Research, 135*(3), 835–868. https://doi.org/10.1007/s11205-017-1571-y

Locke, J. (1988). In P. Laslett (Ed.), *Two treatises of government*. Cambridge University Press. (Original work published 1689).
Marmot, M. (2010). *Fair society, healthy lives: The Marmot review*. University College London.
Maurya, S. K. (2020). A reply to Louis P. Pojman's article "the case against affirmative action.". *Conatus—Journal of Philosophy, 5*(2), 87–113.
Maurya, S. K. (2021). The concept of justice in reference with philosophies of Plato and Aristotle: A critical study. *Journal of Liberty and International Affairs, 7*(3), 250–266. https://doi.org/10.47305/JLIA21370250m
Maurya, S. K. (2022). On just, justice and distributive justice: A critical and comparative discourse. *Journal of Liberty and International Affairs, 8*(2), 240–254. https://doi.org/10.47305/JLIA2282240m
Maurya, S. K. (2024). African philosophies of justice and equity: A contemporary discourse. *African Journal of Religion, Philosophy and Culture, 5*(2), 61–78. https://doi.org/10.31920/2634-7644/2024/v5n2a4
Maurya, S. K. (2025). Restorative justice and karmic justice: Ubuntu and Vedanta in dialogue. *African Journal of Religion, Philosophy and Culture, 6*(2).
Merry, S. E. (2011). Measuring the world: Indicators, human rights, and global governance. *Current Anthropology, 52*(S3), S83–S95. https://doi.org/10.1086/657241
Michalos, A. C., & Land, K. C. (2018). Replies to our commentators. *Social Indicators Research, 135*(3), 1057–1078. https://doi.org/10.1007/s11205-017-1550-3
Nagel, T. (1991). *Equality and partiality*. Oxford University Press.
Nozick, R. (1974). *Anarchy, state, and utopia*. Basic Books.
Nussbaum, M. C. (2006). *Frontiers of justice: Disability, nationality, species membership*. Harvard University Press.
Nussbaum, M. C. (2011). *Creating capabilities: The human development approach*. Harvard University Press.
Plato. (1991). *The Republic* (A. Bloom, Trans.). Basic Books.
Porter, M. E., Stern, S., & Green, M. (2014). *Social progress index methodology report*. Social Progress Imperative.
Rawls, J. (1971). *A theory of justice*. Harvard University Press.
Rousseau, J. J. (1973). *The social contract* (M. Cranston, Trans.). Penguin Books. (Original work published 1762).
Ruggeri, K., Garcia-Garzon, E., Maguire, Á., Matz, S., Huppert, F. A., & Bakolis, I. (2020). Well-being is more than happiness and life satisfaction: A multidimensional analysis of 21 countries. *Health and Quality of Life Outcomes, 18*, Article 192. https://doi.org/10.1186/s12955-020-01423-y
Sandel, M. J. (2009). *Justice: What's the right thing to do?* Farrar, Straus and Giroux.
Sen, A. (1985). *Commodities and capabilities*. North-Holland.
Sen, A. (1999). *Development as freedom*. Oxford University Press.
Sen, A. (2009). *The idea of justice*. Harvard University Press.
Stiglitz, J. E., Sen, A., & Fitoussi, J.-P. (2009). *Report by the commission on the measurement of economic performance and social Progress*. Commission on the Measurement of Economic Performance and Social Progress.
UN. (2015). *Transforming our world: The 2030 agenda for sustainable development*. United Nations.
UNDP. (1990). *Human development report 1990*. United Nations Development Programme.
UNESCO. (2021). *Global education monitoring report 2021/2: Non-state actors in education*. UNESCO Publishing.
Veenhoven, R. (2000). The four qualities of life: Ordering concepts and measures of the good life. *Journal of Happiness Studies, 1*(1), 1–39. https://doi.org/10.1023/A:1010072010360
WHO. (2008). *Closing the gap in a generation: Health equity through action on the social determinants of health*. Commission on Social Determinants of Health, World Health Organization.

Wilkinson, R., & Pickett, K. (2009). *The spirit level: Why greater equality makes societies stronger*. Bloomsbury Press.
Young, I. M. (1990). *Justice and the politics of difference*. Princeton University Press.
Young, I. M. (2000). *Inclusion and democracy*. Oxford University Press.
Ziegler, F., & Schwanen, T. (2011). Transport and social exclusion: A justice-based approach. *Transport Policy, 18*(4), 567–574. https://doi.org/10.1016/j.tranpol.2011.01.011

Chapter 2
Theoretical Foundations of Justice

Justice and the Question of Foundations

The conception of justice, prior to being the subject of social and political philosophy, has been framed within the mythic, ritual, and religious consciousness of archaic societies. Whether due to the shift toward logos or as a result of it, justice, the transition from mythos to logos, transformed justice from a a divine command or social instinct and became a concept that was open to rational investigation and normative evaluation. This development was more than a change in approach: it implied a paradigm shift in justice ontology and epistemology. Justice was given a personification in the mythic consciousness as Nemesis, Dike, or Maat as an embodiment of cosmic and social order. In philosophical discourse, beginning with the pre-Socratics and culminating in the classical dialogues of Plato and Aristotle, justice became both a metaphysical principle and a political telos (Lloyd, 2016). What is important about justice as a foundational notion in philosophical inquiry is not its porous nature in traditions, but the dual nature of a regulative ideal and an evaluative framework that it possesses. As Plato's Republic suggests, justice is not merely a desirable trait among others but the very condition under which other virtues, wisdom, courage, and temperance, can be harmoniously ordered (Plato, 1997, pp. 433a–444e). Plato's metaphysical hierarchy, wherein the Form of the Good illuminates all other forms, situates the idea of justice within an ontological scheme in which knowing and being are bound by rational social order. The justice, understood in this way, is neither contractual nor functional, but rather necessary, unchanging, and objective.

This Platonic move has its detractors, including most prominently those who would position justice not in forms that transcend their context but in contextually circumstanced discourses. Nevertheless, even these criticisms assume that justice has epistemic baggage, that it is a notion, the meaning and use of which demand strict defense. As John Rawls puts it, "justice is the first virtue of social institutions,

S. K. Maurya, *Exploring Justice as a Social Indicator of Life*, Social Indicators Research Series 92, https://doi.org/10.1007/978-3-032-10812-8_2

as truth is of systems of thought" (Rawls, 1971, p. 3). Justice is often compared to truth, which makes the argument that just as societies, like belief-systems, cannot just be evaluated by the outcomes they deliver, but, instead, by what can be justified out of them. Epistemologically, it means that any given narration of justice should not only be normatively plausible but it also should be conceptually coherent, logically integrated, as well as be able to be publicly intelligible.

In addition to its metaphysical and epistemological aspect, justice is anchored in moral commitments central to philosophical reflections. What does it mean to treat others with justice, fairness, and equal moral regard? Does justice regulate itself on the basis of equality, dignity, merit, need, or any combination of the above? These are not just a set of hypothetical questions, but these questions generate the moral terrain upon which human beings bargain over rights, obligations, and chances of life. As Nussbaum asserts, justice must be understood as constitutive of human flourishing, as enabling persons to exercise capabilities essential to a dignified life. This perspective differs with narrow positions of instrumentalism that comprehend justice as an instrument of political stability or economic efficiency. However, justice is that concept by which meaning is ascribed to the institutional frame, as well as to interpersonal relations, that which not only defines how the goods themselves should be distributed, but the structure of recognitional character of personhood as a whole. This ground-level position of justice however posits certain normative tensions, especially between universality and particularity. Normative universalism, as exemplified in Kantian deontology, posits justice as a rational ideal that applies a priori to all rational beings (Kant, 1996). By contrast, communitarian and postcolonial theorists emphasize the contextual, historical, and cultural embeddedness of justice claims (MacIntyre, 2007; de Santos, 2014). What seems right to justice in one polity might be rightly dismissed as oppression in another, bringing into question what the universal norms can possibly mean to their translatability, and their legitimacy. This contradiction is especially high in the globalized world where one conception of justice, be it liberal, Islamic, socialist, or indigenous can turn into a manner of epistemic violence.

The tension cannot be settled without complexity and careful normative consideration. On the one hand, failure to adhere to universality may lead to ethical relativism, on the other hand, an authoritarian adherence to it may result in ideological imperialism. The fundamental question should therefore be reorganized: whether justice is universal or particular does not make sense anymore, but how universal statements about justice can be justified in a manner that does not lose sight of pluralism and power. This entails a second-order reflection on the criteria for moral justification, whether they should be procedural (Habermas, 1996), capability-based, or grounded in mutual recognition. Despite such differences, however, justice, in this sense, works both as ground and as horizon: it provides the basis in terms of which normative evaluation occurs and yet as a horizon relative to which social criticism and institutional redesign must aim. It requires clarity of concepts and lacks abstraction, power of norms, but does not degenerate into dogmatism. Then, as a foundational category, justice is not merely prior to policy but also trans-constitutive of the very possibility of justifying policy, and by extension of being able to make a philosophically meaningful judgment about quality of life (QoL).

Ancient Philosophical Conceptions of Justice

There is nothing in the Platonic corpus to justify the idea that justice is either the doctrine of legal ordering or the problem of distributive arithmetic. Instead, Plato defines justice as a form of harmony as an ontological and metaphysical order first within the soul and in the city. In the Republic, justice (dikaiosyne) is the condition in which "each part performs its own function and does not interfere with that of another" (Plato, 1997 Republic, pp. 433a–434c). At the individual level, this involves the tripartite soul, reason, spirit (thumos), and appetite, being ordered under the guidance of rational judgment. It finds its political reflection in the three-fold organization of the city: rulers, auxiliaries, and producers, with each stratum following its good role. In this scheme justice has nothing to do with adjudication of claims between persons who stand equal with one another but with upholding the status quo of a justly ordered whole. It is a form of ontological balance, a condition of psychic and civic harmony in which the whole is made superior to the parts. Plato's justice is thus radically holistic and teleological, oriented toward the realization of the Good, which is itself the ultimate form and cause of all intelligibility and value (Plato, 1997 Republic, pp. 508e–509c).

The metaphysical richness of the Platonic conception means that it does not resemble contemporary procedural and distributive theories. Justice, here, is neither a contract nor a calculation but an imitation of the cosmos, a metaphysical alignment of the soul and city with the transcendent order of the Good (Annas, 2000). The just man is, we might say, a miniature of the just state, the state corresponding itself to the metaphysical order of being. Yet this vision raises significant philosophical and political questions. Does such a conception allow it to meet the requirements of democratic pluralism? The assumption in Plato model is an essentialist anthropology that individuals are born with natural dispositions, which are matched to the societal roles, philosopher-kings, warriors, and artisans. This metaphysical determinism underwrites a rigid hierarchicalism that stands in tension with modern ideals of autonomy, equality, and democratic participation.

Furthermore, through the establishment of justice as transcendent alternative, as opposed to deliberative concurrence, Plato arguably relegates the intervention of human action in the creation of normative orders. Critics from the liberal tradition have thus viewed the Platonic ideal not as a model for political justice but as a blueprint for authoritarian rule masquerading as harmony (Berlin, 2013). However, the focus on internal order, rational integration, and the Good as the ultimate cause of justice on the part of Plato is a philosophically fruitful addendum to atomistic and instrumentalist theories of justice that were widespread in modernity. In contrast to the metaphysical and macrocosmic perspective of justice proposed by Plato, Aristotle offers a more pragmatic, civic, and anthropological perspective of it. In the Nicomachean Ethics, justice (dikaiosyne) is described not merely as a virtue among others, but as "complete virtue in relation to others" (NE V.1, 1129b30–1129b33). It is the virtue par excellence owing to the fact that it comprises the entirety of the ethical life, which people live in the polis. Both universal and particular, justice is concerned both with lawful action in general and differentiates between distributive and corrective justice.

The principle of distributive justice deals with the division of honors, riches, and other distributable commodities among people based on merit, which is usually thought of as proportional equality. In contrast, corrective justice functions to restore equilibrium in cases of voluntary and involuntary transactions, rectifying injustice by neutralizing gain and loss (NE V.2–4). These distinctions foreground Aristotle's commitment to teleology: justice is intrinsically tied to the function (ergon) of human beings as rational and political animals. This teleological disposition is further seen in the imagination of Aristotle of the organic state of the polis. Unlike contractualist views that see political society as an artifice for mutual gain, Aristotle argues that the polis exists "by nature" (physei), and its purpose is the realization of the good life (eudaimonia) (Politics I.2, 1252b27–30) (Aristotle, 1998). In this case, justice does not act as the limit on the political; instead, justice is the purpose of the political association.

At the heart of the Aristotelian perspective is the concept of proportionality to which Aristotle takes to another level in the sense that proportionality became not only a mathematical but also a moral concept. In justice, unequals must be treated differently, but should be subjected to a proportional degree of equality or inequality, to be based on merit or desert. Nevertheless, Aristotle is not blind to the shortcomings of strict proportionality. His doctrine of equity (epieikeia) functions as a corrective to the universality of legal norms, allowing for the spirit of justice to prevail when literal application of the law would result in injustice (NE V.10, 1137a31–b14). This foreshadows current jurisprudential discussions of the connection between legal positivism and moral reasoning. However, Aristotle's justice is not without normative ambiguities. The issue of what they count as merit in their distributive schemes is not spelt out clearly and it remains historicists, which raises the issue of whether their Game might be susceptible to aristocratic or oligarchic entrenchment. Moreover, Aristotle's reliance on the teleology of the polis excludes those deemed incapable of attaining eudaimonia, namely, women, slaves, and non-Greek "barbarians," thereby undermining the universal scope of justice. Nevertheless, the virtue-theoretic approach of Aristotle is still a great contribution to the philosophical perception of justice despite such limitations. His vision of justice as a personal moral virtue on the one hand, and a structural organization toward the good life on the other hand, simultaneously fills the divide between ethics and politics, the individual and institution, law and equity. His model offers a dynamic account of justice as practical wisdom (phronesis) actualized in communal life, a vision that still resonates in contemporary debates on civic republicanism, capabilities, and the moral purposes of law.

The Early Modern Turn: Contract, Reason, and Rights

The origins of the modern world and the evolution of the idea of justice are deeply intertwined, reflecting the development of political, philosophical, and social structures throughout history. The development of contemporary philosophical conceptions of justice started with a terribly fundamental shift in philosophical thinking about justice established once the Enlightenment. The object of justice was no longer to have a based-route in the intrinsic purpose of the polis itself or in the ethical character of the citizen but was instead reformulated as related to the will of individuals, natural law, and contract. This theoretical discontinuity is one that came about with the emergence of early modern states, decay of feudal hierarchies, and the intellectual turmoil of enlightenment. Its logical shift of justice as virtue to the justice of law, especially as civil law based on consensual authority, was the focus in the reasoning of Hobbes, Locke, and Kant. Both these thinkers reacted to the issues of political power and foundations of legitimate compulsion, attributing, however, varying metaphysical and normative commitments.

Thomas Hobbes's *Leviathan* (1651) posits the modern conceptualization of justice by relocating its origin from nature to artifice. According to Hobbes, there is no justice in the state of nature, for in that pre-political condition, there exists no common power to enforce covenants (Hobbes, 1991, Ch. 13). In the absence of the sovereign, people are in a constant state of mutual insecurity, and are bound by rules of nature, of which self-preservation is the prime rule. As he famously declares, the natural condition is one of war, wherein life is "solitary, poor, nasty, brutish, and short" (ibid., p. 84). To Hobbes, justice involves the fulfillment of bargains, and such bargains only come to have force by reason of the coercive power of the state through the Leviathan, the Leviathan is their sovereign made by covenant. In that respect, justice is radically unnatural: it is not an outcome of human nature but of the dogmas established by an authority situated in the center of the ensemble, to the end of the civil peace. This position satisfies deep discontinuity of the classical tradition where justice precedes and defines political existence. For Hobbes, by contrast, justice is derivative, its existence is contingent upon the institutionalization of power. Yet, Hobbes's theory is beset by enduring philosophical challenges. His insistence on moral minimalism, that justice consists merely in keeping one's contracts under duress of enforcement, seems to strip justice of its ethical substance. Furthermore, the absolute authority of the sovereign, as dictated by the need of order, evokes the risk of authoritarianism. As critics such as Locke and Rousseau would later argue, Hobbes's theory risks reducing the citizen to a subject, denying the reciprocity and moral agency necessary for true political legitimacy. However, Hobbes is more of a forerunner: he locates security, consent, and coercion in the center of modern political thought, grounding the central connection between justice and institutional power.

Unlike the pessimistic anthropology of Hobbes, John Locke gives a more optimistic and morally enriched explanation of the state of nature. While acknowledging inconveniences in the absence of civil authority, Locke maintains that individuals are governed by a law of nature discernible through reason, which teaches that "no one ought to harm another in his life, health, liberty, or possessions" (Locke, 1988, II.6). It is a natural law through which are grounded a set of rights considered inalienable, prior to the state and limiting its legitimacy: life, liberty, and property. According to Locke, the defense and enactment of these rights is justice. The social contract isn't one stipulating of Justice alone, but provides justice on the basis of legitimate authority and rule of law. The paradigm locus of the Lockean justice is property, in particular. Through labor, individuals mix their work with nature, thereby acquiring ownership rights, a process Locke sees as justified by the natural law and necessary for human flourishing. Locke further goes on to present the right of a rebellion, where he states that political authority is justified only to the extent that it upholds the rights of citizens. Should a government violate this compact, the people have the right to overthrow it, a concept that would profoundly influence revolutionary political theory, from the American Declaration of Independence to liberal constitutionalism.

At the same time, proto-capitalist rationale behind Lockean justice has attracted criticism. Locke explains why labor and consent-based property was such a great basis of the right to privately accumulate and market economies. However, this liberal conception tacitly favors possessive individualism and naturalizes socioeconomic inequalities. Moreover, Locke's silence on colonial expropriation and slavery reveals the limitations of his universalism, exposing the ambiguous moral boundaries of the liberal tradition.

Nevertheless, the integration of the natural law, limited government, and individual rights by Locke has been an essential part of contemporary understandings of justice, especially with liberal-democratic theory.

Immanuel Kant reconfigures justice not as a product of fear (Hobbes) or self-interest (Locke), but as the rational expression of moral autonomy. According to Kant, justice pertains to the rightful relations among persons in the external world, relations governed by universalizable maxims and the demand to treat all rational beings as ends in themselves (Kant, 1996, p. 37). The categorical imperative is then transposed into the realm of rights and duties, and becomes justice, the juridical form of it. In contrast to Hobbes and Locke, Kant does not ground justice in empirical desires as well as conventions established in the course of history, but he bases it on practical reason. The moral law, contained within the rational will, places an obligation on a person to act in accordance with principles in a way that can be willed as a universal law. The role of justice in this paradigm is not that of a contract but a deontology one; there is no authority in the consequences but in that the form of the law is the way of its authority. Kant distinguishes between ethical duties (which concern internal motives) and juridical duties (which govern external actions). The latter constitute the domain of right (Recht), and their central principle is that each person's freedom must coexist with the freedom of others under a universal law (ibid., p. 24). Based on this, justice implies the equal liberty of everyone, not just because it is a social construct, but because it is a moral aspect of being a rational agency. The centerpiece of Kant's theory is the vision of a person as dignity: rational beings have a certain dignity, which extends their normative status in limiting how they can be treated irrespective of contingency facts. This moral anthropology provides the foundation for modern conceptions of human rights, constitutional law, and cosmopolitan justice (Habermas, 1996).

Nonetheless, this formalism has been criticized as abstract, relative to historical injustices and social situation, by Kant. Critics argue that by focusing on universal form rather than material substance, Kantian justice may fail to engage with structural inequalities or particular harms. Nevertheless, the autonomy and dignified status of persons emphasized by Kant provide a strong alternative to consequentialist and instrumentalist explanations, making justice rest on the intrinsic moral position of human kind.

Liberal Egalitarianism and Its Discontents

The justice theory developed by John Rawls represents a peak point in the political philosophy of the twentieth century. Rawlsian liberal egalitarianism, which came into being as a reaction to utilitarian orthodoxy and libertarian minimalism, redirected normative theorizing toward concerns of fairness, equality, and the moral autonomy of individuals placed within just basic structure. His theory was both an attempt to revive normative political theory and to find a way of reconciling the ideal of liberty with substantive equality by the means of a theory based on reason, contract, and reciprocity. However, despite its wide influence, Rawls's theory has engendered sustained critique, ranging from concerns about its abstraction and proceduralism to its neglect of power, history, and cultural specificity. These criticisms form the heart of a broader challenge to liberal egalitarianism's claim to normative universality.

In *A Theory of Justice* (1971), Rawls develops a conception of "justice as fairness," rooted in a hypothetical social contract designed to identify principles of justice that free and equal persons would agree to under fair conditions. The central methodological device is the original position, a thought experiment in which rational agents choose principles of justice behind a veil of ignorance, deprived of knowledge of their personal characteristics, social status, natural talents, or conception of the good (Rawls, 1999). The veil promotes neutrality, given that it removes morally arbitrary benefits and forces the contractors to choose principles that are defensible to everyone. From this device, Rawls derives two principles of justice: (1) the principle of equal basic liberties for all citizens, and (2) the difference principle, which permits social and economic inequalities only if they benefit the least advantaged, alongside fair equality of opportunity. These are lexically prioritized principles with the emphasis placed squarely on the liberty above the distributive considerations. This leads to a theory that aims at honoring individual freedom without perpetuating unfair power and opportunity inequalities through constitutional forms. Rawls complements this framework with the notion of public reason, introduced more explicitly in Political Liberalism (1993). In a pluralistic society marked by "reasonable disagreement," justice must be grounded not in a single comprehensive doctrine but in principles that all citizens can accept as free and equal persons (Rawls, 1999). Stability for the right reasons thus becomes a critical desideratum: just institutions must be stable not through coercion or habit, but through the informed allegiance of reasonable citizens (ibid., p. 140). The moral architecture proposed by Rawls is a combination of the Kantian deontology, social contract approach, and democratic liberalism, which is aimed at offering a stable foundation of collaboration among equals under the circumstances of profound moral and cultural diversity. Nevertheless, this is the aspiration that has been criticized not only by the representatives of liberal tradition but those belonging to its outskirts.

Rawls has received criticism on his theory basis despite its decency and normative aspiration because they are too abstract, especially on the person characterization or the use of procedural devices. A main complaint has focused on the so-called unencumbered self, the rational chooser completely free of social, cultural, or historical definition, upon which the original position runs. Critics such as Michael Sandel argue that this conception of the self is ontologically thin, severing moral reasoning from the embeddedness of human agency in traditions, communities, and affective ties (Sandel, 1998). The agents that Rawls, as he phrases it, are antecedently individuated, and hence cannot discern any obligations that are not freely chosen, which constitutes justice to a mutual contractual benefit instead of moral solidarity. Closely related is the critique of proceduralism, that Rawls's method prioritizes fairness in the design of decision-making procedures at the expense of substantive engagement with the historical and material conditions of injustice. This concern is most powerfully articulated by Charles Mills, who in *The Racial Contract* (1997) and *Black Rights/White Wrongs* (2017) challenges the presumption of racial neutrality embedded in liberal contract theory. By bracketing historical realities of slavery, colonialism, racial exclusion, etc., Mills argues that the bold theory of Rawlsian Rawlsian obscures the structural character of injustice. As Mills (2017) puts it, *"the ideal-as-ideal model often has little to say about how we got here or how we get out."* This criticism has also been executed on the epistemology of ignorance claiming that liberalism is based upon a narrow view of political reality but not worldviews of subalterns. According to Mills and other critical race theorists, justice should consider historical constitution of political subjects as well as the asymmetrical condition of epistemic power, to which Rawls veil of ignorance is silent.

Feminist philosophers have raised parallel concerns. Susan Moller Okin (1989) argues that Rawls's model fails to interrogate gendered hierarchies, particularly the division of labor within the family and its impact on the life prospects of women. Rawls unintentionally authorizes an organization of unpaid work and dependency that contravenes the norms of objectivity and mutuality by treating the family as a kind of institution not subject to justice. Similarly, Iris Marion Young (1990) critiques the distributive paradigm of justice as overly individualistic, neglecting the structural and cultural dimensions of oppression, such as marginalization, domination, and misrecognition, that shape lived experiences of injustice. From a postcolonial perspective, scholars such as Bhikhu Parekh (2000) and de Santos (2014) critique liberal egalitarianism for its epistemic parochialism, its tendency to universalize Western values and political norms while ignoring non-Western conceptions of justice. The Rawlsian model presupposes a neutral public space where people act as equal moral agents, and this neutrality, in its turn, is based upon accepting or marginalizing other different worldviews, as they claim. The inability to appreciate the plurality of traditions of justice, that by Islam, Confucian, and indigenous, leads Rawlsian liberalism to accusations of being culturally imperialist. These criticisms bring to bear a critical question regarding the Rawlsian project: was it possible to place liberal egalitarianism on a new footing that takes into some account the normative role of history, the intricacy of self-identity, and the variances of justice demands without compromising a belief in equity and universality? Some scholars, including Nussbaum and Amartya Sen, have attempted to answer this question through the capabilities approach, which shifts the focus from the distribution of primary goods to the real freedoms individuals have to pursue lives they value. An alternative response to this ideal theory is suggested by others, who argue in favor of nonideal theory, a theory of justice that starts with injustice, and puts strong weight on feasibility, reformation, and historical context.

Justice Beyond the Liberal Canon

Even at its most egalitarian articulations, the liberal tradition is constrained by a set of ontological and epistemic assumptions, which have received protracted questioning by a number of philosophical quarters; such assumptions being individualism, procedural rationality, and universalism (Land & Michalos, 2018). The ability to meet the challenges of liberal justice has been under fire among communitarian, feminist, and postcolonial critical thinkers who have not only critiqued the sufficiency of liberal justice but also its very structure and composition with regard to the assumptions it poses about the neutrality of the liberal self, emphasis laid by the liberal justice on distributive paradigms, and parochialism in understanding of moral reasoning by underlying Eurocentric analysis. These interventions do not fill in the liberal canon but attempt to remake the cartography of morality according to which theories of justice are elaborated. Today, there are three principal streams within such critiques.

Communitarian Reorientations

The starkest point of the communitarian criticism is a rejection of moral atomism, which equates individuals as self-sufficient, pre-social agents whose identity and values exist prior to social contexts. Liberal theories, particularly those grounded in Kantian and Rawlsian thought, are said to rely on a conception of the self that is "unencumbered" by history, community, and tradition (Sandel, 1998). This abstraction, though intended to promote impartiality and fairness, has been attacked on the ground that it detaches moral thinking about the real conditions of human agency. According to Michael Sandel, such a model of self does not pass the test of ontological plausibility and normative richness. In place he then posits a situated self, formed by the communal practices and embedded within webs of meaning and commitment. Justice, then, cannot be specified independently of the constitutive ends that emerge from communal life (ibid., pp. 150–166). The liberal appeal to neutral principles beyond substantive conceptions of the good is therefore regarded as philosophically empty and politically fruitless. Alasdair MacIntyre advances this critique in *After Virtue* (1981), where he argues that modern moral discourse has become incoherent, precisely because it has lost the teleological and narrative unity that anchored classical ethics. To MacIntyre, the self is not a single chooser, but a narrative individual, whose being is saved in historically situated forms of practice traditions. Justice, then, is not a case of the application of decontextualized principles but is a case of life well-lived in the practices of a tradition. He proposes a return to Aristotelian virtue ethics, where justice is internal to forms of life that shape human flourishing (eudaimonia). The communitarian turn accepts the rights and the procedural fairness but it demands that the norms have their moral authority vested in moral ecology of communities. It provides a relational account of justice that disputes liberalist tendency to merely use universal processes that are independent of moral content.

Feminist Philosophies of Justice

The epistemological exclusions of liberal justice have been critiqued by feminist theorists as well as the androcentric presuppositions of liberal justice. Carol Gilligan, in her groundbreaking work *In a Different Voice* (Gilligan, 2016), identified a distinction between an "ethic of justice," characterized by rights, rules, and impartiality, and an "ethic of care," rooted in responsibility, empathy, and relational context. She contended socially established theories of moral development favored male styles of moral reasoning and discounted the moral intelligibility of care. The feminist approach to justice should consider more than rights and rules to be just; the voice of the mutual textures of human existence should also be heard. Further continuing on this, Iris Marion Young goes ahead to conduct a broad criticism of the distributive paradigm of justice. In Justice and the Politics of Difference (1990), Young argues that the liberal focus on the allocation of goods obscures the structural and cultural dimensions of oppression—domination, marginalization, exploitation, powerlessness, and cultural imperialism. She argues that justice needs to be rethought on the principles of group differentiation, inclusion, and voice instead of homogeneity and assimilation. Her narration marks the beginning of a move toward a shift related to the distributive justice into the politics of relational justice based on structural change, difference, and recognition. Nancy Fraser, in dialogue with Young and Axel Honneth, advances a dual-dimensional theory of justice that integrates redistribution and recognition (Fraser, 2000). For Fraser, socioeconomic inequality (maldistribution) and cultural misrecognition are analytically distinct but often co-implicated in the reproduction of injustice. The third dimension, participatory parity goes as the normative core: justice demands everyone have access to participate in social life in equal terms. This shift undermines Rawlsian emphasis on primary goods and shifts justice in the direction of institutional positioning that facilitates effective agency. Feminist narratives include criticizing the liberal ignoring of the nonpublic world, and the female and care work in particular, but they additionally rearticulate epistemology: who is legitimate in determining justice, based on which perspective, and with what terms of membership. The feminist philosophy broadens the moral universe of political thought by identifying justice to be embodied and relational and affective.

Postcolonial and Global Justice Perspectives

Bringing into the forefront the geopolitical and epistemic exclusions that are inherent to the liberal canon are postcolonial and Southern epistemologies. Although liberalism claims to provide general models of justice, the same is achieved at the expense of cultures that are not Western by silencing and assimilating normative standards. The postcolonial criticism is not merely about inclusion but about decolonization of the moral and political thought. The capabilities approach given by Amartya Sen offers an especially good illustration of a post-liberal rearrangement of justice. *In Development as Freedom* (Sen, 1999) and *The Idea of Justice* (Sen, 2009), Sen rejects transcendental institutionalism and argues for a comparative framework focused on the real freedoms individuals have to lead lives they have reason to value. According to Sen, justice does not consist in the determination of the ideal institutional arrangements but in the elimination of unfreedoms and the amelioration of capability sets. This system emphasizes the values and plural agency and contextually sensitive inferences, questioning not only utilitarianism and Rawlsian idealism. However, justice is not a destiny of integration within the currently existing liberal framework but an upheaval, a revolutionary advent—a project of ontological liberation. This is a political as well as a self-construction by way of repatriation of self, dismembered by colonial oppression, and internalized inferiority. Gayatri Chakravorty Spivak, in her seminal essay “Can the Subaltern Speak?” (Spivak, 1988), interrogates the discursive mechanisms through which subaltern voices are rendered inaudible in Western epistemic frameworks. To Spivak, justice should come with epistemic accountability: an answerability to all the complicities of knowledge dispersal and hierarchies that suppress or distort marginalized subjects. Boaventura de Sousa Santos goes beyond and establishes a theory of cognitive justice: the right to other epistemologies to coexist and contribute to the creation of a public reason. In Epistemologies of the South (2014), Santos critiques what he calls epistemicide—the systematic erasure of indigenous, popular, and non-Western knowledge by the hegemonic canon of Western modernity. In this context, justice becomes a pluriversal enterprise: not an instance of a unitary rational rule, but the bargaining between multiple normative and cognitive orders. The perceptions of post-colonialism therefore recreate the understanding of justice as global, epistemic, and historical. They insist upon the cessation of mono-logical universalism of liberal theory and avow the polyphonic, dialogical, and decolonial application of normative reasoning.

Justice and Human Flourishing: Virtue, Capabilities, Recognition

The contemporary philosophy of justice has tended to focus on issues of distribution, rights, and institutional authority. However, this more recent philosophical line of thought, still ringing in the ears, considers justice not only as an external rule or order, but also as an internal virtue, not just of individuals, and their relationship with each other, but of institutions themselves, that is, what makes possible the circumstances of human flourishing. However, unlike the paradigm of proceduralism and contractualism, this typology reinstigates the normative role of character, dignity, recognition, and capability as the central components of a good life. In situating justice within the horizon of human flourishing, more contemporary theorists like Martha Nussbaum and Axel Honneth can be said to update classical virtue theory to a modern key, and at the same time they frame it in critique of material deprivation and social misrecognition. This strategy offers a multidimensional view of justice, which incorporates agency as being in constant co-constitutive relation with relationality, and institutional form as a co-constitutive triadality of a just society.

Justice as a Virtue of Social Institutions and Persons

This reorientation has as its critical conceptual starting point the Aristotelian legacy, which was eclipsed in the period of the hegemony of modern liberalism. Aristotle conceived justice as the "complete virtue" (Nicomachean Ethics, V.1, 1129b), manifest both in individual action and in the structures of the polis. The concept of justice on this perspective is not merely about the fair spread of outward goods but rather about formation of character inclined to the common good. The just person acts not from fear of punishment nor mere contractual duty, but out of an internalized disposition to give each their due in a way that sustains the eudaimonic order of civic life (Aristotle, 1999). Modern virtue theorists have attempted to apply this insight to the contemporary institutional background. To them, justice is a normative attribute of institutions, and is not explicable as interpreted on the results or procedures of that institution but rather as a consequence of the virtuous nature of the practices, standards, and end of the institution. As MacIntyre argues, institutions can be evaluated according to their capacity to sustain internal goods—those values intrinsic to human flourishing—rather than simply maximize external goods such as wealth or power (MacIntyre, 2007). In that way, a fair institution does not mean a just one that can only follow just procedures, but one that can contribute to the moral and intellectual growth of individuals.

Nussbaum's Capabilities List as an Index of Just Arrangements

On Aristotelian lines, Martha Nussbaum proposes a capabilities approach to justice as a substantive theory of justice, based on the principle that a just society should guarantee every person the practical ability to live a life that is worthy of dignity as a human being. Unlike utilitarian or resource-based metrics, capabilities theory focuses on what individuals are actually able to do and to be—their substantive freedoms (Nussbaum, 2000). Nussbaum identifies a list of central human capabilities, including life, bodily health, practical reason, affiliation, and control over one's environment, which she argues must be guaranteed up to a threshold level for justice to be achieved (ibid., pp. 78–80). Most importantly, these functionalities are not purely instrumental to human flourishing but are defining features of human flourishing. Justice then is not a merely abstract procedural state of affairs but an actual, material, relational accomplishment, and one accomplished with the aid of social institutions that both foster and safeguard such key functioning. Justice is not an ancillary to education, health care, legal recognition, and environmental sustainability, but prerequisite to the latter. As Nussbaum argues, "a nation that short-changes its citizens in terms of their capabilities is not just poor or inefficient; it is unjust." The capabilities approach opposes the arbitrariness of preference satisfaction theories, and the thinness of formal equality, instead providing a normatively rich and culturally attentive model of justice, which is attentive to embodiment, vulnerability, and dependency. Notably, it also supposes the gender-sensitive lens, in which care work, emotional development, and reproductive freedom are important, defining dimensions of justice, which is usually sidelined by liberal accounts.

Axel Honneth on Recognition and Moral Injuries

In a complementary yet distinct register, Axel Honneth's theory of recognition reconfigures justice around the moral grammar of social relations, emphasizing that injustice often manifests as forms of misrecognition—humiliation, invisibility, or exclusion—that impair individuals' capacity to see themselves as worthy agents. Honneth identifies three spheres of recognition: love (intimate relations), rights (legal personhood), and solidarity (social esteem). Each corresponds to a dimension of personal identity and self-realization, and the denial of recognition in any of these spheres constitutes a moral injury that hinders flourishing (Honneth, 1996, pp. 92–95). The redistributive theories diverge with the approach used by Honneth because the intersubjective conditions of selfhood are the aspects attended to by Honneth. According to this perspective, justice is not predominately concerned with goods, but justice, what it means to be recognized as a bearer of rights, a member of society, and a producer of common good. Institutions are just to the extent that they create spaces for mutual recognition, thereby fostering the conditions under which individuals can develop a practical relation-to-self marked by confidence, autonomy, and respect (ibid., p. 169). The paradigm is particularly relevant when realms of injustice that cannot be reduced to economic ones have to be addressed, i.e., racism, homophobia, ableism, and cultural erasure. These are not merely distributive failures but violations of dignity, experienced as distortions of one's identity and social standing. The recognition theory is therefore in line with feminist and postcolonial discourse, which mainly focus on the affective and symbolic aspects of justice.

The Interdependence of Agency, Dignity, and Material Conditions

These converging lines of thought produce, however, what I will call a relational ontology of justice wherein the relationality of agency and dignity with material conditions is deep and comprehensive. Agency is not an abstract property of the rational chooser, as in liberal contract theory, but a socially embedded capacity—one that must be nurtured by institutions of care, recognition, and material provision (Benhabib, 1992). Dignity is also not just a legal or moral category but an experience, one that is conferred by society and guaranteed by existential flourishing. The capabilities approach and recognition theory leave naked the case of distributive justice as an independent perfection. They critically insist upon a plural and multidimensional approach whereby the notion of justice can be viewed as the development of circumstances in which individuals can present themselves before themselves and others as equality participants in a common moral world. These models overlap too in the thinking that injustice is not just deprivation, but also the deformation, deformation of the self, deformation of the social relations, and deformation of human potential. Within this thickened normative setting, the work of justice is no longer one of distributing goods or of safeguarding entitlements, but of promoting social, psychological, and institutional environments in which flourishing lives may be led. In this sense it is virtue and structure, ideal and practice not, of course, only rigor, but imagination is demanded by philosophy.

Methodological Questions: Ideal Versus Nonideal Theories

It is a well-known fact that the philosophical project of theorizing justice is also faced with the following serious methodological dilemma: How should justice be theorized, as an ideal norm to be striven toward, or as a practical guide under a set of nonideal social circumstances? It has since become one of the thorniest and more important debates in contemporary political philosophy in this divide, which has been framed variously as the question of so-called ideal vs. nonideal theory. One side consists of thinkers (Immanuel Kant and John Rawls), among others, who maintain that normative principles must be generated independently of contingent empirical facts; the other, a swelling group of realist, critical, and postcolonial theorists, musters the claim that an account of justice that does not take historical, political, and practical possibility into account threatens to be morally irrelevant to a point of actually constituting an injustice.

The Aspirations and Limits of Ideal Theory

In its most influential articulation, ideal theory seeks to articulate principles of justice under idealized conditions—where background institutions are just, agents comply with principles, and social cooperation is feasible (Rawls, 1999). Rawls contrasts the ideal theory with the theory of partial compliance and he argues that only through specification of principles of justice that would apply to a well ordered society we can have the clarity as to what exactly justice demands. Ideal theory in this sense serves as a moral ruler, the abstract appraisal criterion against which the nonideal may be gauged and redirected. The roots of this approach can be traced to Kant's moral philosophy, which insisted on the priority of the "right" over the "good," and which required that maxims be universalizable irrespective of circumstance (Kant, 1996). To Kant, justice should be based on pure practical reason, free of empirical characteristics that could corrupt clear moral awareness. Similarly, Rawls insists that ideal theory is not utopian but realistic in the sense that it assumes compliance by agents motivated by a "sense of justice" and institutions that are "workably just" (Rawls, 1999. Yet its critics believe that this form of theorizing about justice, because of its construction of a distance between injustices of the real world, can reinforce both epistemic and moral blindness. Charles Mills calls this "ideal-as-ideal theory" and charges it with constructing moral norms in a "whitewashed" vacuum—ignorant of slavery, colonialism, patriarchy, and structural racism. He contends that Rawls's original position, with its veil of ignorance, is not a neutral heuristic but a theoretical erasure of the historical conditions that shape moral agency and institutional design (Mills, 2017). The main methodological critique, however, is not just that ideal theory is unrealistic, but rather that it is normatively misguided: in its starting point of a fiction of justice, ideal theory may obscure the way that injustice, in the real world, plays out in a systematic and a persistent manner (Maurya, 2025).

Nonideal Theory: Realism, Historical Specificity, and Institutional Critique

To address this perceived abstraction of ideal theory, nonideal theorists have contended that, instead of working with a hypothetical, contract-like relationship between rational agents, normative reflection should start with the felt experience of injustice, as embedded in the historical and institutional context. Amartya Sen (2009) insists that justice must not be formulated solely as a blueprint for an ideal society but as a comparative project: "The theory of justice has to be evaluated in terms of how it helps in addressing questions of injustice in the real world" (p. ix). Central to this more empirical approach, Sen stresses the deprivation with regard to capability, social choice, and the reasoning of the public. The realist vein, based on the works of such theorists as Bernard Williams and Raymond Geuss, is in addition critical of the moralistic or excessively principled approach to politics. Williams argues that political theory must begin from "the first political question"—the securing of order, safety, and trust—rather than from a moral ideal (Williams, 2005, p. 3). On this account justice is not a timeless ideal but an accidental feature that has been produced by negotiation, power, and historical struggle. Geuss (2008) likewise warns against the "ethics-first" model of justice, advocating for a genealogical and critical method attentive to power relations and institutional dynamics. This turn to nonideal theory is not merely pragmatic, but epistemological and ontological. It does not regard injustice as marking a diversion into nonideality, but rather as defining the world, as something that, therefore, any theory must contend with right at the beginning. It turns justice away out of the metaphysical into the political, out of the transcendental to the immanent.

The Demands of Justice in Imperfect, Unjust Societies

The methodological controversy comes to sharp point particularly when we face the normative demands of justice in a context of deeply rooted injustice. Does the justice demand changes in institutions before we can talk about individual accountability? Are the standards of morality that apply to the victims of systemic oppression the same as those to oppressors who enjoy it? Elizabeth Anderson (2010) proposes a "democratic egalitarianism" rooted in the real-world struggles of disadvantaged groups. Justice, to her means, not merely just distributive action, but the overthrow of unjust, that is, oppressive, social relations that impose unequal ranking. Similarly, Iris Marion Young's structural injustice model stresses that injustice arises not from individual wrongdoing, but from normal operations of social institutions, and thus requires collective responsibility and political action (Maurya, 2024). This insistence on structure and shifts in power moves the moral burden away from ideal compliance toward responsible engagement. Then the question arises how to go about normative demands in those cases where all possible options are compromises, where commitment to principle may be the path to inaction, not to change.

How Should Philosophy Engage with Empirical Realities?

The methodological variance of ideal and nonideal theory nevertheless leads to a more fundamental question: What is the place of philosophy in political life? Does it have to express eternal norms, or does it have to interfere in history struggles? Can it do both? Some, like Nancy Fraser (2009), advocate a dialectical model, where normative critique and empirical analysis co-constitute each other. Philosophy should not lose normative aspiration and should not lose its responsibility to material and social contexts of political life. This demands immanent critique, i.e., the criticism of institutions not in comparison with some external ideals but on terms internal to their own practices and their own discourses. Others have claimed that philosophy needs to decolonize itself no longer standing guard against plural epistemologies arising in subaltern and indigenous traditions. Engaging empirical realities thus entails not only empirical attention but epistemic humility—a willingness to unlearn Eurocentric norms of abstraction and neutrality (de Santos, 2014). The approach to justice here should be reflexive, interpersonal, and reparative a practice placed within ongoing processes of critique, solidarity, and change. It has to contend with the violence of the present, without denouncing the imagination of the possible.

Justice, Structure, and Systemic Power

Traditionally, the liberal tradition in political philosophy has been concerned with justice as an end of individual activity and institutional design. However, although this custom has been able to provide valuable insights concerning procedural fairness, liberty, and distributive equality, it has the problem of abstraction of the structural conditions that give rise to and recreate injustice. Conversely, an emerging normative literature has demanded that the question of justice requires the consideration of structural aspects of power, ideology, and institutional entrenchment that maintain social hierarchies and marginalization.

Structural Injustice and the Limits of Individual Blame

Conventional liberal conceptions of justice are inclined to understand injustice as resulting out of discrete wrongful activities of individuals, a violation of rights, breach of contract, or unequal distributions. But this kind of paradigm is inadequate in the face of instances of structural injustice: harms which occur not through the faults or bad will of specific individuals, but through the workings of a system. Iris Marion Young, in her seminal work Responsibility for Justice (Young, 2011), distinguishes between liability models of responsibility and social connection models. The former is concerned with the attribution of blame or responsibility to those individuals who are deemed to have broken overt moral or legal standards. The latter, more structurally attuned model, emphasizes that individuals are implicated in systems of injustice by virtue of their participation in social processes—such as housing, labor, education, or consumption—that cumulatively produce inequality (Young, 2011, pp. 95–122). Notably, this model is not intended to determine the blame but rather develop future responsibilities with an objective of change. The injustice contained in structure thus threatens the ontology itself of the moral subject assumed in much liberal thought. It focuses on interdependency, positionality, and collective entanglement rather than independent agents-making solitary decisions. Moral and political responsibility, then, would no longer be a question of retribution but solidarity and institutional reformation.

Ideology and the Reproduction of Unjust Social Orders

In the sense that structural injustice defines the outer form of direct political power, ideology is the inner logics of it—its cognitive framework. The Marxist tradition (see below) has suggested that ideologies are used to make power natural by making contingent social arrangements appear natural or obligatory. According to Louis Althusser, ideology operates not merely at the level of false belief, but through institutions, rituals, and practices that interpolate individuals as subjects of existing power structures (Althusser, 2001). The schools, media, religion, and also the law become ideological state apparatuses to shape consciousness and limit the horizon of political imagination. This insight is deepened in Gramsci's notion of hegemony, which designates the cultural and moral leadership exercised by dominant groups through consent rather than coercion (Gramsci, 1971). The concept of justice, in terms of such a construction, cannot become limited to the procedural neutrality and distributive fairness; there is a need, via that construction, to also question the normative validity of the social order and the means through which the agreement is fabricated. The justice struggle can then also be defined as a struggle over meaning—which knowledge is considered, which values become institution, and which histories not forgotten.

Contemporary theorists such as Fraser (2013) and Fricker (2007) extend this critique into the realm of epistemic injustice, where ideology distorts not only material relations but also the conditions under which subjects are recognized as knowers. The idea of misrecognition developed by Fraser puts its emphasis on the nature of the relationship between the primacy of the culture (representing domination) and the secondary of the economy (representing subordination), contributing to the social underrepresentation on the level of subordination with both material and symbolic bonds. Fricker's account of testimonial and hermeneutical injustice underscores how marginalized groups are often denied epistemic credibility or the conceptual tools to articulate their experiences—another axis along which systemic injustice operates (Maurya, 2021).

Intersectionality and Systemic Complexity

A critical supplement to structural and ideological critique is the framework of intersectionality, first developed by Crenshaw (1989), which challenges the unidimensional categories often used in justice discourse—race, class, gender—as analytically insufficient. Intersectionality insists that injustice must be understood as multivalent and interlocking, where systems of oppression (e.g., patriarchy, white supremacy, capitalism) mutually constitute and reinforce one another. Philosophically, this calls into question the adequacy of Universalist theories of justice that claim neutrality while assuming an unmarked (often white, male, bourgeois) subject. As Patricia Hill Collins (2009) argues, knowledge and morality emerge from standpoints situated in social structures, and any theory that ignores such positionality risks reproducing domination under the guise of abstraction. Intersectionality is one thing that makes it difficult to diagnose injustice and prescribe remedies. Justice thus stops being an issue of correcting one axis of inequality but rather an issue that aims at changing the matrices in which various types of exclusion are running. This requires a methodological shift toward relational, context-sensitive, and dynamic approaches to justice—what Crenshaw calls an "analytic sensibility" rather than a fixed category (Crenshaw, 2011).

Moral Responsibility Under Oppressive Structures

What comes through as one of the most exasperating philosophical questions posed by structural analysis is the nature of moral agency in situations of domination. How is it possible to blame people who are being exposed to injustice systematically? Is it possible to move freely in unjust systems or are we only carriers of roles and positions that are defined by social forces? Philosophers such as Bernard Williams (1981) caution against attributing full moral responsibility to agents acting under constraints, while others such as Sally Haslanger (2012) argue that recognizing one's complicity in oppressive structures is itself a precondition for agency. The problem is the development of a model of responsibility that is not paralyzed by a sense of systemic determinism on the one hand, or a kind of moralism that places victim-blame on structural circumstances outside his or her control. The notion of collective responsibility becomes central. The similarities between Young social connection model, Fricker epistemic agency, and participatory parity by Fraser all gravitate on the thinking that justice should compel one to make context-sensitive action not as a solitary moral ethic but rather as a member of communal institutions and dialogues. It is not only to purge oneself of complicity, but to practice repair, resistance, and reconfiguration. It should be understood that justice is a praxis, as much as it is an ideal that also needs to be considered historically, critically reflective, and politically active. It does not just require that we dream some new world is possible but that we know how the one we have is operating with all of its complexity and contradiction and embeddedness.

Cosmopolitan and Transnational Justice

The issue of justice can no longer be delimited to the finite aspect of the nation-state in a world that can be characterized by transnational interdependence, global mobility, and systemic inequalities between and among nations. The theorists of cosmopolitan and transnational justice have criticized the normative sufficiency of domestic-centered theories by questioning whether justice principles have to apply to all human beings regardless of whether they belong to other nations. The shift requires a fundamental reconsideration of sovereign authority, duty, identity, and distributive justice, which lays a particular emphasis on the moral and political relevance of global systems in proselytizing life opportunities.

Liberal theories, most notably that of Rawls in The Law of Peoples (Rawls, 1999), have often accorded moral significance to national boundaries, asserting that principles of justice apply primarily among conationals who share a political culture and institutions of reciprocity. Rawls distinguishes between "peoples" and "states" and argues that a "society of peoples" ought to be governed by principles of mutual respect, nonaggression, and basic human rights, rather than full distributive justice across borders (Rawls, 1999, pp. 23–25). In the case of Rawls, the obligation to help only involves getting "burdened societies" just institutions, but not distributive equality. It has been claimed by critics that this statist commitment of justice is both morally arbitrary, and also normatively unresponsible. Provided that nationality is not relevant to moral worth of people as Rawls himself argues in the domestic case of justice, it is unclear why Rawls should need to bracket moral worth at the border. Charles Beitz, in Political Theory and International Relations (Beitz, 1979), rejects this internal/external bifurcation, contending that the same moral principles that govern distributive justice domestically must apply internationally, especially in light of global interdependence (Beitz, 1979, pp. 129–132). According to Beitz, the relationship of interdependence in a global economy is institutionalized to the extent that the Rawlsian criterion on the basic structure applies to the global arena. Consequently, international inequalities cannot be treated merely as unfortunate and natural facts, but are the product of systems in which the global wealthy are fully integrated, and to which they draw systemic advantage (Maurya, 2020).Among the strongest statements of global distributive justice is the work of Thomas Pogge, a development of the Rawlsian moral theory that accuses global institutional structures of promoting poverty and inequality through their operations. In World Poverty and Human Rights (Pogge, 2002), Pogge argues that affluent societies are not merely failing to help the global poor—they are actively harming them by imposing and maintaining a global order that institutionalizes unjust patterns of wealth and power.

Pogge unveils the theory of a so-called negative duty: the duty not to sustain coercive order that sustains deprivation. The present global market, in the sense of its trade regulations, indebtedness structures, and protection of properties, clearly fails this responsibility by means of systematically excluding the world poor out of the outcomes of growth. He contends that even a minimal commitment to justice would require structural reform of global institutions, such as fairer trade agreements, global taxation mechanisms, and enhanced regulatory capacities (Pogge, 2002, pp. 197–204). This argument would make global poverty not an unfortunate accident, but a perversion of structural violence, so the main responsibility is not just the manifold venality of local elites, but it is in the very design of global governance. It also tackles liberal voluntarism, which sees obligations to be brought about through express agreements or a common nationality, by the notion that by taking part in hurtful orders even, one can create duty.

Even though cosmopolitanism holds that all people have equal moral status, its institutional and normative implications are controversial. Kantian cosmopolitanism, as articulated in Perpetual Peace (1795), envisions a federation of free republics governed by international law and a shared respect for universal rights. Kant's ideal of cosmopolitan right includes the right to hospitality and nonhostile treatment of foreigners—anticipating modern refugee ethics and global human rights (Kant, 1991, pp. 105–108). Contemporary cosmopolitans such as David Held and Daniele Archibugi have advanced the idea of cosmopolitan democracy, which seeks to democratize global governance by expanding accountability, participation, and justice beyond the state (Archibugi, 2008; Held, 1995). They champion that the current international institutions like UN, WTO, and IMF have a democratic deficit because they uphold the interest of elite and lock away the poor in all the world into nonrepresentational areas. Nonetheless, cosmopolitanism has been criticized as a too thin view of identity and overreaching in terms of norms. Michael Walzer, in Spheres of Justice (Walzer, 1983), argues that distributive obligations are morally thick only within bounded communities united by shared meanings and history. To Walzer, justice is a culturally specific entity, and the idea of universal validity is prone to offend the autonomy of local customs. Similarly, Chandran Kukathas (2003) warns against the imposition of global norms that may override plural values and communal self-governance. This critique is echoed in postcolonial perspectives, which caution that cosmopolitanism may become a civilizing discourse, veiling global power asymmetries in the language of universal justice (de Santos, 2014). With the struggle between the cosmopolitan moral universalism and the nationalist or pluralist allegiances we have to ask: are we able to formulate a cosmopolitanism of the bottom: one that can accommodate diversity and hold the power of the globe accountable?

Despite their differences in normative assumptions and political strategies, theories of transnational justice have common points in the necessity of global institutional transformation. Thomas Pogge is an institutional cosmopolitanist whose approach emphasizes negative obligations and international institutional architecture. He calls for innovations such as the Global Resources Dividend, a tax on the exploitation of global resources redistributed to the global poor (Pogge, 2002, pp. 196–201). In contrast, David Held gives weight to democratic legitimacy and procedural inclusion in the global decision-making process. His model envisions a multilayered governance structure where sovereignty is shared among local, national, and global bodies, each subject to accountability and the rule of law (Held, 1995, pp. 92–107). Charles Beitz develops a version of pragmatic cosmopolitanism, he does not accept the form of abstract idealism, but nevertheless acknowledges the moral imperative to establish global justice. He contends that cosmopolitan justice must be sensitive to contextual pluralism while insisting on equal moral worth as the regulative ideal (Beitz, 1999, pp. 146–163). As a combination, these theorists help to define the various aspects of global justice, namely, institutional design, normative justification, democratic participation, and historical critique. I do not see any consensus developing but I do see what is at stake: in a world being characterized by worldwide movements of capital, labor, goods, and information, justice has to broaden its vision to that of the moral geography of globalization.

Concluding Summary

When understood as free of monolithic desirable models, the philosophical inquiry into justice discloses a topography of normative approaches: the procedural, the distributive, the aspect of recognitions, and the aspect of relations, each bringing into view and foregrounding a modality of ethically permissible human flourishing and social order. By the above discussion, it can be concluded that no theory can exhaustively without remainder the moral greatness or the institutional requirements of justice. Rather, what is morally needed is a multi-plural not integrated conception, one that achieves both normative coherence and normative criticality, one that does not fall into reductive universalism and yet escapes into relativism but one that maintains rigor and avoids collapsing into relativism. This form of conception should be both theoretically detailed and practically involved, so as to connect the philosophical conceptualization of justice and its outward manifestation.

It is interesting to note that an account that would be comprehensive of justice must include these historical forms of justice. Procedural justice, classically emphasized by John Rawls and Habermas, concerns the fairness of decision-making processes, the transparency of institutional norms, and the impartiality of legal and political procedures (Maurya, 2022). Distributive justice, from Aristotle through contemporary egalitarianism, focuses on the allocation of primary goods, opportunities, and burdens in accordance with merit, need, or equality (Nussbaum, 2011). Recognitional justice, emphasized by theorists such as Axel Honneth and Nancy Fraser, addresses the symbolic and affective dimensions of injustice, how individuals and groups are seen, valued, or mis-represented within social relations (Fraser, 2000; Honneth, 1996). The relational aspect additionally supports the notion that justice cannot be reduced to transactions or distributions but lies in the way the relationship is structured: among individuals, among citizens, and citizens and institutions, or between peoples beyond borders. As Elizabeth Anderson (2010) argues, "the point of equality is not sameness but the elimination of social relations of domination and subordination." That means that justice is the state of affairs where people can consider one another as equals in the moral status, the legal status, the status of being an agent in participation (Maurya, 2022). These dimensions are conceptually distinct but normatively intertwined. Non-substantive equality by its own procedural fairness dangers legitimating structural inequalities; identity recognition with no transformation in material circumstances can reify without changing alienating relationships; care about social solidarity that fails to be redistributive can reproduce alienation. In this way, justice needs to be viewed as a multidimensional norm, with several axes, none of which can be dispensable in the just society (Michalos & Land, 2018).

Noticeably, any nonideal conception of justice should avoid the temptation to reduce apparently many normative considerations to a single master principle. Although, Kantian deontology, utilitarianism, and Rawlsian contractarianism possess intuitive internal rationalities, by making them exhaustive, they threaten normative reductionism. Justice as experience and aspiration cannot be measured by any unitary measure or constitution axiom. As Amartya Sen observes, "the pursuit of justice is not about achieving the perfect, but about removing remediable injustice." The rationale, then, is to come up with a normatively ontologically integrative, but not totalizing, framework. Interesting to mention a model is what Nancy Fraser (2009) calls a "three-dimensional theory of justice," encompassing redistribution, recognition, and representation. The second one is Martha Nussbaum's capabilities list, which offers a modular, non-hierarchical architecture of human entitlements. Both theories can be viewed as a shade of universalism: both have normative claims that transcend contexts but are receptive to cultural specificity and democratic dialogue. This is neither eclecticism nor relativism; it is a pluralist methodological stance, which allows recognition of the multidimensionality of human experience and multiplicity of moral views. It establishes that justice has to speak the language of the universe but has to be sensitive to the languages of locality of sufferings, dignity, and aspiration.

The issue of pluralism veers very close to relativism, particularly in multicultural or indeed postcolonial scenarios that imply that the establishment of global norms can be subject to epistemic imperialism. However, it's opposite, cultural isolationism, damages justice as an urgent necessity. The task is to hold open a space for cross-cultural ethical dialogue, where norms are not imposed but argued for, revised, and contested in light of shared human experiences and overlapping moral vocabularies (Appiah, 2006). Philosophical engagement must therefore be intercultural, reflexive, and dialogical. As de Santos (2014) argues, justice must be plural not only in its moral content but also in its epistemological sources—engaging indigenous, feminist, Southern, and subaltern knowledges as legitimate participants in the construction of global norms. It is the justice that not only listens but legislates, and one that not only reasons but silences not, and one that does not efface in universalizing. Such a project requires what Miranda Fricker (2007) calls epistemic justice: the fair distribution not only of goods and rights, but of credibility, authority, and interpretive resources. In its absence, justice is reduced to a reverberating chamber of dominating voices, a professional order that cannot question its omissions.

The philosopher of justice is, lastly, made to reconcile the profession of analytic abstraction with the political urgency. There must be a conceptual clarity to prevent the drifting toward moral obfuscation or rhetorical indeterminacy. However, clarity should not be at the expense of normative urgency, or the appreciation of the fact that justice is not just a contemplative virtue but instead it is a public requirement. Philosophy has to face the world of pluralistic unfairness and controversy and transform it by providing insight into how the world is, and how it could be. This is the twin mission of justice, to diagnose wrongs that exist and to fantasize other arrangements. As Iris Marion Young (2011) reminds us, "the point of justice is not only to guide institutions, but to motivate agents to confront injustice in all its forms." It is in this spirit that the plural and integrated conception of justice is not a definitive response but discloses itself as a continuing investigation that keeps critical thought, respects human dignity, and seeks to reckon with the changing contours of global life. It is a philosophy-based theory, with an application in the field of social action, which resides in refection yet is pointed toward transformations.

References

Althusser, L. (2001). *Ideology and ideological state apparatuses*. In *Lenin and philosophy and other essays*. Monthly Review Press.

Anderson, E. (2010). *The imperative of integration*. Princeton University Press.

Annas, J. (2000). *Platonic ethics, old and new*. Cornell University Press.

Appiah, K. A. (2006). *Cosmopolitanism: Ethics in a world of strangers*. W.W. Norton.

Archibugi, D. (2008). *The global commonwealth of citizens: Toward cosmopolitan democracy*. Princeton University Press.

Aristotle. (1998). *Politics* (C.D.C. Reeve, Trans.). Hackett Publishing.

Aristotle. (1999). *Nicomachean Ethics* (Terence Irwin, Trans.). Hackett Publishing.

Beitz, C. (1979). *Political theory and international relations*. Princeton University Press.

Beitz, C. (1999). Justice and international relations. In *Political theory and international relations* (2nd ed.). Princeton University Press.

Benhabib, S. (1992). *Situating the self: Gender, community, and postmodernism in contemporary ethics*. Routledge.
Berlin, I. (2013). *The power of ideas*. Princeton University Press.
Crenshaw, K. (1989). Demarginalizing the intersection of race and sex. *University of Chicago Legal Forum*, 139–167.
Crenshaw, K. (2011). Twenty years of critical race theory. *Connecticut Law Review, 43*(5), 1313–1322.
de Santos, B. S. (2014). *Epistemologies of the south: Justice against Epistemicide*. Routledge.
Fraser, N. (2000). Rethinking recognition. *New Left Review, 3*, 107–120.
Fraser, N. (2009). *Scales of justice: Reimagining political space in a globalizing world*. Columbia University Press.
Fraser, N. (2013). *Fortunes of feminism: From state-managed capitalism to neoliberal crisis*. Verso.
Fricker, M. (2007). *Epistemic injustice: Power and the ethics of knowing*. Oxford University Press.
Geuss, R. (2008). *Philosophy and real politics*. Princeton University Press.
Gilligan, C. (2016). *In a different voice: Psychological theory and women's development*. Harvard University Press.
Gramsci, A. (1971). In Q. Hoare & G. Nowell Smith (Eds.), *Selections from the prison notebooks*. International Publishers.
Habermas, J. (1996). *Between facts and norms: Contributions to a discourse theory of law and democracy* (W. Rehg, Trans.). MIT Press.
Haslanger, S. (2012). *Resisting reality: Social construction and social critique*. Oxford University Press.
Held, D. (1995). *Democracy and the global order: From the modern state to cosmopolitan governance*. Stanford University Press.
Hill Collins, P. (2009). *Black feminist thought: Knowledge, consciousness, and the politics of empowerment*. Routledge.
Hobbes, T. (1991). In R. Tuck (Ed.), *Leviathan*. Cambridge University Press.
Honneth, A. (1996). *The struggle for recognition*. MIT Press.
Kant, I. (1991). In H. Reiss (Ed.), *Political writings*. Cambridge University Press.
Kant, I. (1996). *The Metaphysics of Morals*. (M. Gregor, Trans.). Cambridge University Press.
Kukathas, C. (2003). *The Liberal archipelago: A theory of diversity and freedom*. Oxford University Press.
Land, K. C., & Michalos, A. C. (2018). Fifty years after the social indicators movement: Has the promise been fulfilled? *Social Indicators Research, 135*(3), 835–868. https://doi.org/10.1007/s11205-017-1571-y
Lloyd, G. (2016). *The man of reason: "Male" and "female" in Western philosophy*. Routledge.
Locke, J. (1988). In P. Laslett (Ed.), *Two treatises of government*. Cambridge University Press.
MacIntyre, A. (2007). *After virtue: A study in moral theory*. University of Notre Dame Press.
Maurya, S. K. (2020). A reply to Louis P. Pojman's article "the case against affirmative action.". *Conatus—Journal of Philosophy, 5*(2), 87–113.
Maurya, S. K. (2021). The concept of justice in reference with philosophies of Plato and Aristotle: A critical study. *Journal of Liberty and International Affairs, 7*(3), 250–266. https://doi.org/10.47305/JLIA21370250m
Maurya, S. K. (2022). On just, justice and distributive justice: A critical and comparative discourse. *Journal of Liberty and International Affairs, 8*(2), 240–254. https://doi.org/10.47305/JLIA2282240m
Maurya, S. K. (2024). African philosophies of justice and equity: A contemporary discourse. *African Journal of Religion, Philosophy and Culture, 5*(2), 61–78. https://doi.org/10.31920/2634-7644/2024/v5n2a4
Maurya, S. K. (2025). Restorative justice and karmic justice: Ubuntu and Vedanta in dialogue. *African Journal of Religion, Philosophy and Culture, 6*(2).
Michalos, A. C., & Land, K. C. (2018). Replies to our commentators. *Social Indicators Research, 135*(3), 1057–1078. https://doi.org/10.1007/s11205-017-1550-3

Mills, C. (2017). *Black rights/white wrongs: The critique of racial liberalism*. Oxford University Press.
Nussbaum, M. (2000). *Women and human development: The capabilities approach*. Cambridge University Press.
Nussbaum, M. (2011). *Creating capabilities: The human development approach*. Harvard University Press.
Okin, S. M. (1989). *Justice, gender, and the family*. Basic Books.
Parekh, B. (2000). *Rethinking multiculturalism: Cultural diversity and political theory*. Harvard University Press.
Plato. (1997). Republic. In J. M. Cooper (Ed.), *Plato: Complete works* (pp. 971–1223). Hackett Publishing.
Pogge, T. (2002). *World poverty and human rights: Cosmopolitan responsibilities and reforms*. Polity Press.
Rawls, J. (1971). *A theory of justice*. Harvard University Press.
Rawls, J. (1999). *The law of peoples*. Harvard University Press.
Sandel, M. (1998). *Liberalism and the limits of justice*. Cambridge University Press.
Sen, A. (1999). *Development as freedom*. Oxford University Press.
Sen, A. (2009). *The idea of justice*. Belknap Press.
Spivak, G. C. (1988). Can the subaltern speak? In C. Nelson & L. Grossberg (Eds.), *Marxism and the interpretation of culture* (pp. 271–313). University of Illinois Press.
Walzer, M. (1983). *Spheres of justice: A defense of pluralism and equality*. Basic Books.
Williams, B. (1981). *Moral luck: Philosophical papers 1973–1980*. Cambridge University Press.
Williams, B. (2005). *In the beginning was the deed: Realism and moralism in political argument*. Princeton University Press.
Young, I. M. (1990). *Justice and the politics of difference*. Princeton University Press.
Young, I. M. (2011). *Responsibility for justice*. Oxford University Press.

Chapter 3
Measuring Quality of Life: Social Indicators Overview

Introduction

The concept of quality of life (QoL) has risen to the status of popular allusion in the public policy, international development, and social science. Broad agreement though this may seem, there is a conceptual wilderness behind it all. So what is this quality life thing? What is the best way to transform conceptions of flourishing, dignity, agency, and justice, so strongly normative in nature, into measurable signs of their philosophical substance? This chapter begins by grappling with this essential dissonance: the desire to render normative ideals empirically measurable without draining them of their moral substance or epistemic texture. The philosophical importance of assessing quality of life is that it tries to unite two historically separate dimensions: the normative, which deals with the question of what ought to be; and the empirical, which deals with what is. In Aristotelian terms, this represents a fusion of phronesis (practical wisdom) with epistēmē (scientific knowledge), necessitating not only technical accuracy but ethical insight. To Plato, justice was not a variable that could be added and subtracted and added again: it was the right ordering of the soul and polis. However, in the present context, justice is confined to policy matrices, dashboards, and developmental indices, wherein the transition necessitates philosophical inquiry.

The Necessity of Operationalizing Normative Concepts

Well-being and justice cannot stay conceptual to make any impact when it comes to institutional design, budgeting by the government, or international governance. However alluringly abstract ideals of morality are, they are inert without translation moves that provide the means of passage between principled reasoning and

S. K. Maurya, *Exploring Justice as a Social Indicator of Life*, Social Indicators Research Series 92, https://doi.org/10.1007/978-3-032-10812-8_3

practical judgment. According to Amartya Sen (2009), one does not need a fully ideal theory of justice to address manifest injustices. Instead, public reason demands that we have evaluative concepts, however provisional, in terms of which injustice can be discerned and corrective action be taken.

The question, therefore, is not whether to measure, but how to measure in an ethical, reflective, and philosophically responsible manner. It does not imply succumbing to the technocratic urge to regard measuring as a strictly technical exercise. Indicators are not neutral representations; they are normative constructions embedded in epistemic regimes, policy imaginaries, and value-laden worldviews (Fukuda-Parr & Yamin, 2017; Merry, 2011). As Ingrid Robeyns (2005) notes in the context of the capabilities approach, the process of selecting dimensions and weights in a metric is not merely methodological but fundamentally ethical and political.

The Challenge of Complex Human Goods

In the middle of the problem of measurement lies the irreducibility of some human goods. Dignity, a sense of autonomy, or relationality cannot be scalarized. They do not have value in discrete magnitudes but in certain qualitative forms of life, which are arranged by history, culture, and affect. As Isaiah Berlin (1969) has shown, the plurality of values entails incommensurability, that is, the impossibility of fully translating one good into another without loss. A life rich in social solidarity but low in income is not necessarily less "valuable" than one defined by material affluence but relational isolation. This attempt at quantifying the quality of life would thus have to find its way through a normative contradiction: to transform qualitative, multidimensional, and culturally relative values into quantitative surrogates without losing their moral understandability. This issue is compounded by the fact that individuals may adapt preferences to oppressive conditions, a phenomenon Sen (1985) refers to as "adaptive preferences." Indicators of such persons, such as subjective well-being, may record excellent levels in individuals who are living in gendered injustice, or long-term poverty due to internalized deprivation. Self-report based measures of satisfaction or happiness run the risk of being epistemically naive, or even complicit in structural injustice. Measurement, therefore, must be attuned not merely to surface-level preferences, but to the normative depth of agency and capability; the real opportunities available to live a life one has reason to value (Nussbaum, 2011).

Epistemological Stakes of Quantification

There are some serious epistemological concerns that occur when reducing human experience to measurable quantities. And what is lost through bringing lived realities into the statistical forms? Whose is put in the construction of the metrics, and whose is left out? These questions, draw attention to what Miranda Fricker (2007) calls epistemic injustice: the denial of credibility or interpretive resources to marginalized knowers. The exclusion of indigenous epistemologies, feminist knowledges/Southern frameworks in indicator design does not entail simply bias but structural silencing. Moreover, indicators often function as what Sally Engle Merry (2011) calls "technologies of governance." They determine what comes into view, what matters most, and what ultimately matters. In a similar respect, indicators do not represent a passive reflection of social reality, but have an indexicality such that they are used as tools of world-making. They are capable of generating political momentum, raising money, and redirecting institutional attention, but they can also conceal injustice through a focus on the quantifiable at the expense of the significant. The demand to present similar, scalable, digestible data can lead to moral minimalism, with only those elements of the quality of life that can be quantified being recognized, and others, like intimacy, trust, and freedom of fear, being ignored or pushed to the periphery.

This does not argue against measurement as such, but with a normative vigilance. To have a place in the project of justice, indicators will have to be built and read in a language of ethical transparency and critical self-reflection. They have to be cognizant of deliberative pluralism, amenable to challenge, and grounded in context-sensitive moral arguments. Otherwise, we endanger reifying an image of justice which is empirically convenient, but normatively vacuous. The quality of life (QoL) measuring project, however, is not simply an epistemic project; it is specifically a moral and political project. It demands exact philosophic negotiation amid the fantasy of universality, the necessity of context, between analytic lucidity, and lived complexity. It does not aim to essentialize flourishing to a figure, but to design a number of resources that would help to perceive injustice, make the muffled voices heard, and guide effective intervention. This chapter shall continue by tracking the intellectual history, methodological approaches, and debates of social indicators of quality of life. By so doing, it will establish a philosophical tenet off of which the notion of justice may in fact be able to be proffered, no longer, however, as a normative finish or consummation, but as an indicator in and of itself, with the prospect of guiding policy, reformation, and shared desire.

Historical Evolution of Social Indicators Research

This fundamental shift in the project of measuring human well-being, now core to environments of public policy, international development, and ethical economics, has been experienced during the last one hundred years of the project. The research community on social indicators has a long history, stretching back to the economic determinism of the early twentieth century (approximately 1900–1930) and encompassing the freeway-inspired program-intensity studies of the 1950s and 1960s through the more multidimensional and normative focus of the modern versions. Behind the seeming neutrality of measurement hangs a contentious approach to epistemology, a response formed under the influences of Enlightenment rationalist science, positivist science, and act-utilitarian morals. The emergence of alternative metrics to GDP, such as the Genuine Progress Indicator (GPI), Human Development Index (HDI), and Multidimensional Poverty Index (MPI), reflects not only methodological refinement but a normative rupture: a recognition that life's value exceeds its economic representation, and that justice and well-being require metrics attuned to plurality, dignity, and capabilities.

In GDP to GPI: Economic Determinism and the Origins of Counter-Metrics

The preeminent measure of national prosperity for most of the twentieth century, Gross Domestic Product (GDP), originated from a wartime context and a narrowly economic vision of social progress. Originally intended neither as a measure of human welfare nor as a comprehensive measure of economic welfare, GDP was initially formally defined by Simon Kuznets in the 1930s and was adopted during World War II. GDP was used to marshal military production and economic planning. Indeed, Kuznets himself warned that "the welfare of a nation can scarcely be inferred from a measure of national income" (Kuznets, 1934, p. 7). However, in spite of these caveats, GDP has ended up dominating the moral imagination of policy-makers as well as international institutions during the middle of the twentieth century. It was so appealing because it was quantifiable, comparable, and universalistic, all of which were features of enlightened rationalism. The unspoken presumption was that, once economic growth was attained, social progress would automatically follow within the context of classic liberal economics, compounded by a technocratic sense of postwar administration. This form of economistic reductionism, however, by the 1970s began to receive increased criticism. The publication of The Limits to Growth (it is a report which examined the implications of exponential economic and population growth in the context of finite global resources) and the Stiglitz-Sen-Fitoussi Report (Sen, 2009) questioned the validity of GDP as a proxy for well-being, highlighting its failure to account for environmental degradation, inequality, unpaid labor, and social cohesion. In response, alternative indices such as the Genuine Progress Indicator (GPI) were developed to adjust economic activity for social and ecological costs. GPI incorporates factors such as income distribution, environmental sustainability, and nonmarket labor, pointing toward a normative recalibration of measurement itself (Talberth et al., 2007). Technical improvement aside, the transition between GDP and GPI encompasses a re-estimation of the philosophical kind: a replacement of aggregative materialism with evaluative pluralism, of economic output with human flourishing as the object of central interest.

The Post-war Welfare State and the Social Indicators Movement

The Social Indicators Movement emerged in the Post-War Welfare State. The Liberal democracies in the Global North embarked on an expansion of welfare systems like never before following the devastations of World War II. This resulted in the desire to have noneconomic indicators, which would track social growth, the performance of institutions, as well as the welfare of the citizenry. In this context, the social indicators movement emerged, most prominently through institutions such as the United Nations, the Organisation for Economic Co-operation and Development (OECD), and later the World Bank and UNDP. The UN's Universal Declaration of Human Rights (1948) offered an early template for multidimensionality, recognizing not only civil and political rights but also social, economic, and cultural rights. Nonetheless, it was hard to translate these normative ideals into working indicators. Early social well-being measurement attempts tended to emphasize education, health, employment, and housing, e.g., the Social Indicators Yearbooks of 1960s/1970s, usually based on welfare economics and the management of government, but still wrestling with conceptual uncertainty. OECD's Social Indicators Programme (initiated in 1971) and later the Better Life Index signaled a more systematic attempt to institutionalize the measurement of noneconomic dimensions of well-being. The goal of these indicators was to give policy-makers evidence-based information on the quality of life, and at the same time be responsive to the concerns of the people, and democratic validity. Nonetheless, even these initiatives revealed tensions between policy-driven simplification and moral complexity, a tension that continues to haunt social indicators today (Noll, 2002). The postwar world, therefore, represented a shift out of unidimensional measures of economic performance into the multidimensional measures of social progress, which were beginning to be seen as rooted in the increased understanding that justice, inclusion, and agency were not incidental consequences of economic growth; they are first-order goals of social development.

Enlightenment Rationalism and Positivist Influence on Measurement

The tradition of social indicators has its philosophical pedigree, in the legacy of Enlightenment rationalism, the view, held through the natural world, too, that not only human affairs, but the natural world as well could be made intelligible through empirical observation and rational abstraction. It is an epistemological stance that, being productive of scientific stringency, established a reductive bias: the presumption that what is morally important must be quantifiable in some numerical way. This rationalist urge was further influenced by the positivism and specifically had Auguste Comte who conceived sociology as the social physics. The hierarchy of sciences advanced by Comte positioned the moral and political sciences toward the end of a continuum that concluded in objective knowledge hence naturalizing the perception that measurement was an objective of intellectual maturity. This yielded a technocratic imaginary in which quantification was equated with objectivity, precision, and neutrality, a view that has been widely critiqued in contemporary philosophy of social science (Cartwright & Montuschi, 2014; Hacking, 1990). In the utilitarian tradition and particularly in the writings of Jeremy Bentham the desire to sum up pleasures and pains opened up a fantasy (an ambition) of the emergence of a hedonic calculus, an arithmetic of human welfare. One of the descendants of Benthams project was prescriptive rather than descriptive and concerns the aggregating of utility across persons and giving rise to economic cost–benefit analysis, welfare economics, and more recently to the subjective well-being metrics. Although such models helped with some preliminary operationalizations of both happiness and satisfaction, they also stripped the rich moral topography of human life down to preferences that were measurable but somehow removed any context, power, and identity. In such a way, the genealogy of social indicators cannot be disconnected with the intellectual history of the Western epistemic power where measurement is not just a descriptive method but the indicator of epistemic legitimacy. As scholars in feminist, postcolonial, and critical theory have noted, such claims to neutrality can mask the normative exclusions and silences embedded in the very act of measurement (de Santos, 2014; Merry, 2011).

Normative Assumptions in Early Social Science Quantification

Early attempts to put human welfare in a quantitative form to build on a veil of objectivity were based indeed on normative assumptions about that nature of the good life, the structure of society, and the purpose of governance. These presuppositions were seldom spelt out, and resulted in what is sometimes called moral naturalism, in which conventional categories and signs were tacitly assumed to be an expression of what is important, but not necessarily what is measurable. In the tradition of Benthamite utilitarianism, the goal of maximizing aggregate happiness presupposed that individual welfare is both separable and summable, a claim that has been vigorously contested by philosophers such as John Rawls and Martha Nussbaum, who argue that rights, dignity, and capabilities are not reducible to aggregate utility (Rawls, 1971; Nussbaum, 2006). The same point can be made of Comtean sociology, which implicitly supported a functionalist concept of society where stability was comparatively synonymous with health and deviance with pathology, wherein normativity is actually incorporated into measurement as a medium of such values. Such frameworks usually presupposed a Eurocentric notion of progress, which consisted of industrialization, secularity, and the nation-state. As de Santos (2014) has argued, such models function as instruments of epistemic imperialism, exporting particular valuations of life under the guise of universality. Rather than simply indicating technical advancement, the history of social indicators research has outlined both a normative and epistemological conflict over the nature and structure of human well-being, and the standards of decency by which to define it, to measure it, and to act upon it. The narrow economism of GDP to the multidimensional indexes of the present day, each one represented more profound philosophical debates concerning the purpose of life, the purpose of a society, and the ethics of knowledge. That indicators should be placed in the service of the cause of justice, it follows that their history should not be conceived as simply a story of innovation, but as a field of critique, a store of assumptions to be questioned and of resources to be reinvented. In this respect, the subsequent passages of the chapter will discuss conceptual underpinnings, methodological approaches, and philosophical debates around the modern-day indicators of social well-being, as a prologue to the future assertion that justice itself is able to be viewed as a social indicator of quality of living.

The Philosophical Foundations of Measurement

The business of quantifying human well-being is fraught with ontological, epistemological, and axiological complications. In contrast to the quantification of natural phenomena, social goods, satisfaction with life, or justice dealings occur in the zone of normative notions, i.e., those whose significance is disputable and culturally informative and normatively loaded. This raises the foundational question: What counts as measurable? To put it more accurately, is it even possible to measure something that is considered qualitative, multidimensional, and something that is evaluatively thick in itself like the quality of life (QoL)?

Ontological Status of Well-Being and Social Goods

With respect to well-being and social goods, this assumption is not clear cut. Unlike physical quantities (e.g., temperature or weight), which refer to observable properties governed by natural laws, well-being refers to evaluative states, situated within normative, cultural, and experiential contexts. Thus, any attempt to define and measure well-being presupposes a moral ontology: a conception of what it means to live well, flourish, or lead a life of value (Griffin, 1986; Scanlon, 1998). Philosophical disagreement begins here. To the hedonists, well-being means pleasure or painlessness. What matters, to the desire-satisfaction theorists, is fulfilment of preferences, regardless of their content. Objective list theories, by contrast, propose that certain goods, health, education, autonomy, relationships, constitute well-being regardless of individual attitudes (Parfit, 1984). All these accounts presuppose a quite various ontology of the good life, and thus more or less accompanying implications of what can and should be measured. The shift to measurement is also even more challenging when social goods are brought into the picture; e.g., justice, equality, or recognition. These are neither rudiments of personal biography, but relational, institutional, and symbolic structures. To measure them requires not only empirical indicators but a theory of social ontology—an account of how institutions, norms, and practices constitute and distribute value (Honneth, 1995; Searle, 1995). Therefore, the quantification of well-being is not only a statistical one, but also a metaphysical and ethical one, rooted in disputable insights as to what does and does not exist and as to what is and is not important.

The Epistemic Tension: Objectivity Versus Subjectivity

The principal input of the quality of life (QoL) measurement is the epistemic clash of objectivity and subjectivity. Should we assess well-being by looking at how people feel about their lives (subjective indicators), or by examining the conditions under which they live (objective indicators)? It is not just a methodological dispute; it embodies more profound philosophical disputes concerning the origins and grounds of evaluative knowledge. Subjective well-being measures, such as life satisfaction scales or affective reports (e.g., "How happy were you yesterday?"), have become widespread in economics and psychology. They are rooted in phenomenological immediacy: the assumption that people are the most qualified to determine what makes them well ordered. However, this dependency of subjective data has been criticized on several bases. First, adaptive preferences may lead individuals to report satisfaction in objectively deprived conditions (Sen, 1985). Second, subjective states are influenced by transient moods, cultural norms, and social desirability biases, undermining their reliability as stable indicators of flourishing (Haybron, 2008). Conversely, objectively measurable criterion, like income, health, education, or housing, might not include the subjective meaning and based experience. An objectively well-provisioned life can also be empty, alienated or not free. Thus, neither pole is sufficient. According to Martha Nussbaum (2011), any serious metric of human development must integrate both objective and subjective dimensions, recognizing that well-being is lived through embodied, reflective, and relational experiences. It is the philosophical work to strike a middle epistemic ground that neither descends into mercury by a relativism of sheer subjectivism nor places the warm blood of objective imposition. This requires many plural methodologies, participatory structures, and it requires, first of all, a measure of reflexive humility regarding the epistemic limitations of any such practice of measurement.

Conceptual Inquiry: "Well-being," "Welfare," "Utility," "Capability," "Functioning," "Life Satisfaction"

In the discourse of social indicators, all the major terms come with varying philosophical baggage. It is important to clarify their meaning to prevent conceptual confusion and normative ambiguity.

- Well-being: Well-being, which is arguably the most general and most disputed term, refers either to subjective happiness, objective flourishing, or integrated states. Its lack of precision is both a strength, enabling interdisciplinary dialogue, and a weakness, inviting equivocation (Crisp, 2013).
- Welfare: The conventional use of welfare, particularly economics, denotes material resources and ability to gratify preferences. However, this approach is vulnerable to preference deformation and market-dependent valuations, often failing to capture deeper ethical concerns such as autonomy, dignity, or recognition (Anderson, 1993).
- Utilitarianism (Utility): central to utility and welfare economics—confuses well-being with desire gratification or satisfaction. While analytically tractable, this reduces normative complexity to a single scalar metric, disregarding qualitative distinctions between goods (Mill, 1861).
- Capability and Functioning: Capability and functioning, introduced by Amartya Sen and Martha Nussbaum offer a more extensive vocabulary. A functioning is a state of being or doing (e.g., being well-nourished, engaging in political life), while a capability refers to the real freedom to achieve various functionings. This approach emphasizes freedom, pluralism, and agency, offering a morally thick and context-sensitive conception of well-being (Nussbaum, 2000; Sen, 1993).
- Life Satisfaction: Life satisfaction is a term that is frequently employed in psychology and survey studies to assess the overall evaluative judgments people hold on their lives. Yet such judgments may be influenced by cultural expectations, momentary affect, or lack of alternatives, raising questions about their normative sufficiency (Diener et al., 1999).

They are not simply terminological variations on well-being of individuals, but are competing visions of human good, each of which is relevant to determining how the quality of life is to be measured and by whom.

The Problem of Value Commensurability: Pluralism and Measurement

The problem of value pluralism is perhaps the most severe philosophical opposition to measurement. As articulated by Isaiah Berlin (1998) and Elizabeth Anderson (1993), many of the values we care about, freedom, equality, community, creativity, love, are incommensurable. They are not meaningfully comparable to a shared yardstick with moral distortion. A society can achieve increased aggregate income, but lose in cultural vibrancy; increased access to education, but also increased inequality. To prioritize such trade-offs on strictly numerical scale is to perpetrate normative violence: to simplify moral complexity of a trade-off to a quantifiable efficiency. This is a complication to standard practices of aggregation and index construction that assumes at least some notion of commensurability or cardinal comparability. Even multidimensional indicators such as HDI depends on implicit weight schemes that hold some few values at higher valuation than others. Although such may be justified on practical grounds, they hide the normative decisions that are ingrained in the architecture of measurement. Sen (1992) acknowledges this difficulty but argues for "incomplete ordering,"the idea that partial, non-comprehensive comparisons can still guide rational deliberation and institutional design. The intention in this case is no longer to resolve the pluralism of value in the false precision but to set up evaluative spaces where pluralism is retained and made observable, albeit not at once in the best order. The epistemic and normative neutrality of measurement can be traced in the philosophical grounds of measurement where no indicator can be epistemically innocent or normatively neutral. Each quantification is a reflective and performative enactment of a series of ontological assumptions, epistemic commitments, and axiological priorities. Measuring well-being is the creation of a normative image of the world, the selection of what is measured, what is apparent, and what is important. This is where philosophy can deliver in a pluralistic world where cultural diversity, structural inequality, and challenged moral terrains are commonplace, this does not mean that it is possible to get rid of this complexity but rather to philosophically engage with this complexity. The practice of measurement needs to be ethical: it must be subjected to criticism, experience-sensitive, and characterized by humility. It is only in such way indicators can be used not as reductions to justice, but instruments of moral imagination and of speaking publicly.

Key Frameworks for Measuring Quality of Life

The mission of quantifying quality of life has spawned a number of competing theoretical approaches, each with a differing conceptual scheme, normative standpoint, as well as methodological framework. These frameworks, ranging from utilitarian subjectivism and capability theory to composite indices such as the HDI and holistic experiments like Bhutan's Gross National Happiness (GNH), differ not only in what they measure but in their underlying metaphysics of the human good, epistemic assumptions, and political purposes. Thus, it is necessary to critically examine the philosophical architecture of four dominant approaches: the utilitarian-subjectivist tradition, the capabilities approach, the human development index and its successors, and novel holistic models including the OECD Better Life Index and the UN Sustainable Development Goals (SDGs).

The Utilitarian-Subjectivist Tradition

At the core of classical and neoclassical economic approaches to well-being lies the utilitarian tradition, which seeks to evaluate states of affairs in terms of their capacity to maximize utility, whether construed as pleasure (Bentham), happiness (Mill), or preference satisfaction (modern welfare economics). Contemporary extensions of this model have focused on subjective well-being (SWB), often measured through life satisfaction surveys and hedonic experience sampling (Kahneman & Krueger, 2006).

Pioneers such as Richard Layard (2005) and Daniel Kahneman and Krueger (2006) have popularized the use of happiness indexes to assess national well-being. These methods normally use high-survey data where people respond on measures of their happiness or contentment on numerical scales. This information is ultimately pooled and compared across populations so governments can monitor the emotional tone of their societies and adjust policy to reflect this. In philosophical terms, utilitarian-subjectivist model presents a philosophic advantage seen in the benefits of interpersonal comparability and empirical easy-openness. It offers as well a unitary gauge of well-being, easily translated into cost–benefit analyses and public budgeting. Yet this strength is also its limitation. The sum total of subjective preferences or inclinations distills away the qualitative variety of human goods down to a question of state of momentary mood or preference, expressed without any context or criticism. Critics such as Amartya Sen (1985) and Martha Nussbaum (2000) have pointed to the dangers of preference adaptation, wherein individuals in oppressive conditions adjust their expectations downward and report high levels of satisfaction. The process of this so-called adaptive preference formation makes clear that subjective satisfaction is not necessarily associated with objective prosperity or ethical fairness. For example, a woman living in a patriarchal culture that has learned to accept norms of subordination might answer that she is very satisfied with life; an inmate who has been subjected to coercive discipline might exhibit consistent psychological stabilities. Thus, subjective data can misrepresent deprivation, legitimating unjust conditions under the guise of contentment (Nussbaum, 2000, pp. 115–116). Moreover, the utilitarian paradigm assumes the commensurability of pleasures and preferences, a notion challenged by value pluralists such as Isaiah Berlin (1998), who argue that some goods (e.g., autonomy, dignity) are qualitatively distinct and irreducible to mere satisfaction. Based on this, the utilitarian measures, though they could be applicable in some of the areas concerning the public health or policy, present an incomplete moral complexion of the well-being, and thus are not fully applicable within a concept measuring the aspect of quality of life.

The Capabilities Approach

The response to utilitarianism limitations and limitations of a resource-based approach has been proposed by Amartya Sen, and subsequently developed by Martha Nussbaum, which took the form of capabilities approach; a normatively rich and philosophically superior model of measuring the quality of life. This approach shifts the focus from subjective states or material possessions to the real freedoms people have to be and do what they value. (Sen, 1999, pp. 18–19). The model revolves around the difference between functionings and capabilities. The functioning is a state that has been reached, i.e., is nourished, educated, or mobile. A capability is the substantive opportunity to do these functionings. In this way, two people who share the same functionings could experience opposite freedom: the former person out of his own free will, and the latter person could be poor.

The capabilities approach thus places agency, choice, and moral autonomy at the center of evaluative reasoning (Nussbaum, 2006). Among the philosophical successes of this paradigm, one can include pluralist ontology: this paradigm does not presuppose a unified measure of good life but rather acknowledges the inextricable plurality of human flourishing. Martha Nussbaum, for example, proposes ten central capabilities such as bodily integrity, emotions, practical reason, and the ability to have control over the surrounding environment. These are not derived from preference or income but from a philosophical anthropology grounded in human dignity and developmental psychology (Nussbaum, 2011). Yet the capabilities approach is not without challenges. There is both methodological and normative difficulty in interpreting philosophical concepts as subject to policy-operable indicators. Which capabilities should be included? How should they be weighted? Can they be measured reliably across cultures? Sen resists prescribing a fixed list, favoring public reasoning and democratic deliberation, whereas Nussbaum defends a universalist list grounded in cross-cultural consensus and moral theory (Nussbaum, 2011, pp. 32–33). The approach has also been cited by critics as a data-intensive, epistemically complex. Capabilities tend to involve counterfactual reasoning: we do not just want to know what people are doing but what they can do, under their constraints and circumstances. This introduces measurement ambiguity and philosophical contestation, especially in societies where information on freedoms, choices, and structural constraints is incomplete or contested (Robeyns, 2005). Nonetheless, the most powerful alternative to utilitarianism has been the capabilities approach that presents a powerful image of justice and well-being, which is the enabling of agency in dignified conditions.

The Human Development Index (HDI) and Beyond

In 1990, under the influence of Sen's theoretical work, the United Nations Development Programme (UNDP) introduced the Human Development Index (HDI) as a composite measure of life expectancy, educational attainment, and per capita income. Though modest in scope, the HDI marked a symbolic break from GDP as the singular measure of national progress, establishing the precedent for multidimensional well-being measurement in global policy (UNDP, 2020). The HDI was created pragmatically in order to provide a crude but conceptually founded measuring method of national ranking. It has three dimensions that indicate capabilities-informed interpretation; longevity as a proxy of health, education as a form of agency, and income as an instrumental good. However, HDI has been criticized for being overly simplistic, arbitrarily weighted, and insensitive to internal inequalities (Klugman et al., 2011).

In response, the Inequality-adjusted HDI (IHDI) and the Multidimensional Poverty Index (MPI) were later developed. These indices disaggregate development viewing deprivation not only in one dimension but take into consideration various facets such as nutrition, child mortality, years of schooling, access to electricity, sanitation, and others. They offer a more nuanced depiction of well-being by acknowledging overlapping forms of disadvantage (Alkire & Santos, 2010). These indices, which retain the instrumental focus of the HDI, philosophically, include elements of the capability theory. However, they are themselves compound indices, built using mathematical forms of normalization, index aggregation, and index weighting, which can hide the value-laden assumptions built in the index design. For example, does a schooling year hold the same moral value in one cultural setting as it does in another? Is power concentrated on access to electricity at expense of political voice or cultural participation? Moreover, even ranking the countries based on such indices can by itself strengthen developmentalist hierarchies and epistemic domination, in which particular patterns of life are considered insufficient by the establishment of externally established criteria. As de Santos (2014) argues, even the most sophisticated indices risk epistemicide—the silencing of alternative worldviews under the guise of universal measurement. In this way, although HDI and its follow-ups are a crucial breakthrough conceptually, their philosophical adequacy can only rely on constant democratic contestation, local manipulation, and epistemic reflexivity.

OECD Better Life Index, Gross National Happiness (Bhutan), and the SDGs

Within recent decades, several holistic models have been developed that have attempted to bring together the psychological, environmental, and cultural aspects of well-being into policy-relevant contexts. The OECD Better Life Index (BLI), introduced in 2011, includes 11 dimensions such as civic engagement, work–life balance, community, and environmental quality. It offers an interactive platform, allowing users to assign weights according to their own values, thus foregrounding individual and cultural variation (OECD, 2011). Similarly, Bhutan's Gross National Happiness (GNH) index, first proposed in the 1970s and formalized in 2008, evaluates well-being across nine domains, including psychological well-being, ecological diversity, good governance, and time use. GNH is grounded in Buddhist ethics, explicitly rejecting materialism and embracing spiritual and collective dimensions of flourishing (Ura et al., 2012). In contrast to technocratic indices, GNH strives to be philosophically embedded and culture based, a challenge to the Western-centric patterns of development.

The UN Sustainable Development Goals (SDGs), launched in 2015, comprise 17 goals and 169 targets encompassing poverty eradication, gender equality, climate action, peace, and justice. Although it is not actually a quality of life (QoL) index, SDGs indicate an all-embracing moral image of the world well-being. However, their sheer breadth and lack of prioritization have been criticized for diluting normative clarity and measurement feasibility (Fukuda-Parr & McNeill, 2019). The normative implication of the presence of these whole frameworks is an influence to decenter economic measurement, plural values, and democratize measurement. Yet they also raise questions about data standardization, cultural translation, and the risk of performative measurement, where indicators serve bureaucratic visibility more than ethical guidance (Merry, 2011). The paradigms examined in this part all stand in making an important contribution to the project of quality of life (QoL) measurement. The utilitarian models are simple and comparative but they lack depth with regard to their morality. Moral depth of capability theory is due to the fact that it faces complication in operations. Composite measurements such as HDI and MPI have institutional pull, though they accumulate the danger of epistemic bias. They give importance on holistic models to incorporate cultural inclusivity, although they have methodological difficulties in terms of coherence and accountability. The philosophical challenge is not to select between these frameworks as mutually exclusive, but to think about the ways in they can and perhaps should be coupled, criticized, and transformed in the face of justice, dignity, and plurality. The challenge is to ensure that measurement is a zone of contestation and normative imaginaries, and not a policy instrumentation exercise. It is only at that point, indicators can be used not as the reductive proxies but as the philosophically defensible means to the furthering of human flourishing.

Critical Perspectives on Quantification and Objectivity

The popularity of quantification, as the device par excellence of epistemic neutrality, scientific objectivity, has a long history. In particular, where public policy and development studies are concerned, the use of indicators, supposedly objective, quantifiable, and universal, has become the holy grail of evidence-based governance. Nevertheless, the ideological, normative, and disciplinary preconditions of quantification have become more apparent as a result of the critical philosophy. Indicators are not only descriptive but quite the contrary, they contribute to the construction, regulation, and normalization of social reality. This idea engages with four prominent critiques: (1) Michel Foucault's analysis of measurement as a function of biopower and governmentality, (2) Pierre Bourdieu's concept of symbolic violence and the imposition of dominant epistemic norms, (3) the critique of model thinness by Nancy Cartwright and Mary Morgan, and (4) postcolonial interrogations of the coloniality of knowledge, which ask: Whose quality of life is being measured, and by whose standards?

Foucault: Measurement as a Technology of Biopower and Governmentality

Michel Foucault's critical genealogies of modern institutions, especially in *Discipline and Punish* (Foucault, 1977) and *The Birth of Biopolitics* (Foucault, 2008), reveal how quantification functions as a tool of governance. Modern power as explicated by Foucault is necessarily not only repressive or juridical but, most importantly, productive. It acts by generating subjects, normalities, and truths using administrative, scientific, as well as statistical machinery. Measurement is central to what Foucault terms "biopower," the control and optimization of populations through demographic knowledge, health indices, census data, and other forms of state rationality (Foucault, 2008, p. 317). According to this perspective, social indicators are not impartial depictions but a method of governmentality, i.e., a way of knowing a population that is coherent and susceptible to intervention. The extensive application of indicators as a process in health, education, and poverty might be seen to be the embodiment of what Foucault has referred to as the conduct of conduct: management of conduct and making conduct visible, comparable, and responsible. The indicators are the markers of normality and abnormality; they are the things worth caring and controlled. Notably, this criticism does not mean that measuring is inherently oppressive. Instead, we should be speaking of a genealogical vigilance: of what kinds of life are opened up, what kinds of lives barred, when we act in the name of the numbers. An illustrating example would be the life satisfaction indexes simply present subjective well-being rather than normalizing specific versions of happiness and pushing the noncompliant versions of human flourishing to the periphery.

Bourdieu: Symbolic Violence and the Epistemic Power of Indicators

Another step building on this critique is provided by Pierre Bourdieu, who demonstrates that indicators play their role in the fields of power, which are governed by symbolic domination. In *Distinction* (Bourdieu, 1984), Bourdieu argued that classification systems, taste hierarchies, academic credentials, income brackets, are not mere reflections of social reality but mechanisms of legitimation. They reiterate classes even as their symbolic differences become incorporated in what seem to be impersonal vehicles of assessment. The idea of symbolic violence was introduced by Bourdieu and it is particularly enlightening in relation to social indicators. The indicators (such as standardized tests or development indices) establish hegemonic cultural and epistemic norms in the name of universality. As an illustration, the undervaluing of traditional education in global indicators of well-being can overshadow the native knowledge systems or informal learning models. The quantification here is a form of misrecognition by which the dominated internalize externally defined norms of value and long to standards not their own. In addition, the institutional inertia of flawed indicators can also be explained with the help of Bourdieu. Once an index (e.g., GDP or HDI) becomes entrenched in policy, funding, or global rankings, it accrues symbolic capital, a kind of epistemic authority that is difficult to dislodge, even in the face of critique. So, the question that Bourdieu forces us to put is simply this: whose values are inscribed in our indicators, and whose it is to determine what is development, education, or quality of life?

Cartwright and Morgan: Models the Slimness of Models and Limits of Quantification

Nancy Cartwright and Mary Morgan, in their seminal work The Philosophy of Economics: Models and Matters of Fact (Cartwright & Morgan, 1999), offer a critique of economic modeling that extends to the domain of social indicators. They contend that models are not transparent windows on to the real world; they are constructed in order to simplify, idealize, and abstract away the complexity. In so doing, they tend to be epistemically weak, they provide measurable deliverables, which conceal assumptions, data gaps, and normative decisions. This is major criticism of composite score indexes such as the HDI, GPI, and MPI. These models are based on normalization formulas, weighting schemes, and indicator selection processes that can be arbitrary or led by institutional convenience other than deliberative judgments putting normative pressure on it. As an example of this thought, equal weights in the HDI given to income, education, and life expectancy implicitly imply a quantification of moral equivalence that is seldom supported by anything other than the blind belief that since the HDI is made up of equal weights they must therefore be morally equivalent. Cartwright warns against the "simulacrum of science"—the illusion that numerical precision implies epistemic authority (Cartwright, 2007, p. 19). Moreover, the philosophy behind many models causes worries in relation to external validity and ontological sufficiency, in terms of the context-insensitivity of such models. What might be an appropriate metric in Norway would not be suited to rural Bangladesh not necessarily because of cultural difference, but because of structural inequalities of power and resources as well as historical progression. In this way, Cartwright and Morgan propose model pluralism, local calibration, and a more humble epistemology, i.e., an epistemology that does not involve models as yardsticks.

Coloniality of Knowledge: Who Measures, and For Whom?

The postcolonial and decolonial theory is perhaps the most incisive criticism of social indicators as it questions the epistemic injustice underlying the global practices of measurement. Scholars such as Boaventura de Sousa Santos, Gayatri Chakravorty Spivak, and Walter Mignolo argue that the global regime of indicators constitutes a form of "epistemic colonialism," where Western norms of development, success, and happiness are exported as universal benchmarks (de Santos, 2014; Mignolo, 2011). This is not just methodological error at risk here but a matter of erasure when it comes to ontology. Insofar as global indicators narrowly describe poverty, education, or health in economistic or biomedical terms, they tend to discredit other lifeworlds, other forms of subsistence economies, nonliterate knowledge forms, and spiritual forms of health and well-being. Indicators thus become instruments of what Spivak (1988) famously called "epistemic violence": the silencing of subaltern ways of knowing. This criticism has far-reaching normative issues: Is it possible to have a universal definition of the good life? Can cosmopolitan indicators be made without rendering cultural and ontological differences flat? The intellectual act of requesting cognitive justice as formulated by Santos requires that said measurement activities be not only multiperspectivist, participatory, and contingent, but also cognizant of epistemic agency of the subjects of measurement. Material consequences such as utilization of participatory processes, qualitative statistics, and story mode in indicator design and political responsibility within international governmental systems such as the World Bank or UNDP are also the aspects of concrete implications. It is not a goal to give up on the concept of measurement, but a decolonial move to transition measurement toward extractive technocracy to dialogical ethics. The criticisms of Foucault, Bourdieu, Cartwright, and postcolonial theorists all boil down to the same point: quantification is not an epistemically neutral act, but rather a normatively loaded, politically important, and epistemically contingent practice. The role played by indicators in the process of subjectivities construction, power reproduction, and the definition of the good life does not depend on their technical or well-intended nature.

To the extent that social indicators should possess the potential to contribute to justice and not to cover it, they need to be reflexive. This implies an acceptance of the fact that they all possess genealogies, cultural preferences, and institutional orientations of the past. It further implies that measurement must be incorporated into the philosophical discourse, active citizenship, and moral responsibility. And in this sense, measuring must not be viewed as a termination of social truth, but as a platform arguable and subject to revision, an opening to communal reasoning, moral speculation, and ethical analysis. It is only under such conditions it can turn indicators into something not of domination but emancipation.

Justice, Distribution, and the Ethics of Indicators

In a world that has become dominated by data, indicators have become core policy planning tools of political decision-making, institutional accountability, and international comparisons. Yet their capacity to open or to close justice is extremely controversial. The indicators are not just descriptive instruments but normative instruments, they count some lives and epistemically ignore other lives. They are designed and used in ways that directly relate to the distributive, recognitional, and procedural aspects of justice, and they create sticky philosophical questions about who is visible, who is listened to, and who is made statistically insignificant. It necessitates to examine four essential issues: (1) indicators as tools of distribution and recognition, (2) the ethical problems of aggregation, (3) the importance of procedural justice and epistemic inclusion, and (4) the role of indicators in public reasoning and deliberative democracy.

Indicators as Distributive and Recognitional Tools

The truth is that in the center of justice stands the question of distribution: resources, opportunities, capabilities, and care. But justice is also about recognition, the acknowledgment of persons and communities as worthy of moral and political regard (Fraser, 2003; Honneth, 1995). The indicators are not only distributive devices but also they work as recognitional tools, and they determine what is measured, who is counted, and whose needs will be prioritized. In case, for example, the choice of whether to include sanitation access, maternal health, and literacy in a national well-being index chooses which domains will have funding and government policy. On the other hand, unquantified areas, such as mental health, indigenous languages, or informal labor, can become invisible, which causes repeated neglect and structural marginality. This is what Amartya Sen calls "informational deprivation," a condition in which people's suffering is not only unaddressed but unseen within the dominant evaluative framework (Sen, 2009). Indicators, then, are ontological validators, in a recognitional way: they highlight the character of moral objects of the state. According to Miranda Fricker (2007), epistemic injustice occurs when individuals or groups are denied the status of credible knowers or are excluded from processes of meaning-making. (Maurya, 2020) In measurement, this is evident when elite technocrats define quality of life for marginalized populations without their input, thereby reenacting what de Santos (2014) calls "epistemicide," the silencing of local knowledge systems.

The Ethical Dimensions of Aggregation

The patterns of aggregation summaries as averages, indices, or composite scores are becoming prevalent interventions to collect and summarize complicated social information. Yet it raises pressing ethical questions. Whose realities are represented in averages? And who disappears in the process? Aggregated data often flatten moral variation. The average income may increase in a country with improving income inequality. A community in which one minority group has systemic discrimination might be drowned in national satisfaction rankings. As Amartya Sen (1992) and Elizabeth Anderson (1993) have both emphasized, justice cannot be inferred from statistical aggregates alone. The risks of aggregation include the danger of what might be called moral compression, the effacement of notable differences in need, in dignity, in vulnerability. Further, there is a normative aspect to index construction, i.e.: which factors should be given more weight? What specific ingredients to use in the case of education versus income, or health versus political freedom. These are never even clear decisions, but the sort of decisions that define global development agendas and internal priorities. Therefore, aggregation is not a morally neutral mathematical process but a right or wrong (in the moral sense), including judgments about what to count, how much, and to whom. This raises the need for disaggregated and intersectional data. As scholars of intersectionality (Collins, 2000; Crenshaw, 1989) have shown, social identities such as race, gender, class, and disability intersect to produce overlapping structures of disadvantage. Averages mask these realities. To measure ethically, one not only has to be concerned with means outcomes but also with differences within and between groups, as well as with the location of the subject within structures of power.

Procedural Justice and Epistemic Inclusion

The fairness of measurement is not only an issue of results, it is also a matter of processes: who plans the indicators, who is involved in their creation, and whose opinions are seriously addressed. Drawing from the work of Miranda Fricker (2007) and de Santos (2014), it becomes clear that epistemic justice, the fair treatment of people as knowers, is crucial in indicator construction. Conventional methods of social indicators tend to depend on expertise that is mostly top down, leaving out the experience of people whose lives they quantify. Not only does this undermine the legitimacy of metrics, this also continues epistemic marginalization. A countercheck to this is provided by participatory modes of working, whether through citizen scorecards, community-based monitoring, or deliberative metric design. They seek to include affected communities in the co-creation of indicators, enabling what Sen (1999) calls public reasoning.

Democratic participation in indicator design serves three philosophical goals:

- Epistemic pluralism: Acknowledging varieties of knowledge, such as experiential knowledge, indigenous knowledge, and narrative knowledge.
- Procedural justice: The absence of a reinforcement of status levels of know-how and exclusion due to the design of metrics.
- Reflective equilibrium: Fostering ongoing dialogue between normative principles and empirical realities (Rawls, 1971).

However, participation must be substantive, not symbolic. It must be inclusive of creation of capacities, redesigning, and true power-sharing. Otherwise, indeed, participatory approaches threaten to become mere window-dressing, which serves to legitimize technocratic domination in the process of pretending inclusiveness.

Indicators as Instruments of Public Reasoning

Indicators have a role beyond just an administrative role in spurring on some sort of public deliberation. Amartya Sen has argued that measurement should not seek epistemic finality, but stimulate critical dialogue about what matters, why, and for whom (Sen, 1993, 2009). According to this concept, indicators should be not absolute rating but fallible stimuli of democratic thought. The indicators considered in this vision are not merely judged on the basis of predictive performance or even aesthetic statistical properties, but in their power to inform moral and political debate. A good indicator asks questions such as why is child mortality increasing in one place? Why is the situation of access to education getting better among boys rather than girls? What forms of inequality are hidden in our data? Indicators turn into discursive artifacts, and not even substitutes to a judgment but rather helps to make one. They encourage the reader, whether citizen, policy-maker, or scholar, to participate in a common vernacular of assessment, which is informed both by empirical evidence and normative value. This role is particularly significant in pluralistic societies where different visions of what constitutes a good life have to be accommodated by each side, operating within the same institutional structures.

Sen's ideal of public reasoning implies that indicators should be:

- Transparent in their construction and assumptions
- Accountable to those they affect
- Revisable in light of new information and critique

This makes measurement a democratic undertaking that is based not on technocratic guarantee but on reflexive modesty and normative openness. As it has been discussed that indicators should not be viewed solely as empirical instruments only, but as moral constructions. They inform our images of justice, our idea of what is valuable, and our manner of political interaction. The ethics of indicators demands that we step out of the technocratic mantle of neutrality and adopt a more philosophically guided approach to the participatory and justice-based manner. It is on this ethical reorientation that we can turn indicators into a source of managerial control and a source of moral visibility, democratic empowerment, and human dignity.

Challenges in Integrating Justice into Quality-of-Life Measurement

With the discourse on human development adopting more and more the language of justice, the question arises whether justice can itself become a social indicator, or whether it empowers the selection, meaning, and application of indicators as a meta-norm. The concept of justice is multifaceted, situation-specific, and normatively dense, and converting it into a quantifiable measure poses a philosophical and methodological conflict. It is one thing to measure it, but it is something more in maintaining moral and political thickness of justice as one moves through the limits of policy instruments. The dangers of conceptual distortion, cross-categorization of similarities and distinctions, e.g., inputs and outcomes, and the proclivities to methodological reductionism cannot be underscored. This lends a potent argument to hybrid methods, which blend accuracy with precision and rigor of the quantitative data, as well as richness of the qualitative data.

Justice as Indicator or Meta-Norm?

Justice holds an ambiguous place in measurement discourse. It is frequently deployed as a normative ideal, a point of reference according to which arrangements in society may be judged, but is increasingly being examined as a variable, susceptible to statistical analysis and to be referenced as a policy benchmark. This dual role raises foundational questions. Is justice to be quantified per se, meaning tangible issues such as the feeling of fairness, trust in institutions, or even access to legal systems? Or could it be measurable indirectly like by proxies that are used like income distribution or health equity or political participation? The other perspective holds that justice is a meta-concept, that is, it is an aspect that delineates the space where the indicators are judged, but it cannot be narrowed down to one indicator. According to this perception, justice cannot be measured as an object, but it is a lens that defines what is supposed to be quantified, how to subdivide data, and in whose voices to incorporate into the design of metrics. Nevertheless, it is quite tempting to use justice as a pointer since policy-makers tend to insist on operating clarity. This may be easier to apply to incorporation of policy but there is a risk that justice by so doing can be deprived of its normative depths (Maurya, 2021).

Disaggregating Justice-Oriented Metrics: Inputs, Outputs, Outcomes, and Capabilities

The process of integrating justice in measurement is sometimes hindered by the lack of distinction between various categories of assessment. The resources involved are called inputs and can include education budgets or health care funds. These are deliverables that are instant, including schools being constructed or the vaccines getting out. The results are quantifiable, e.g., literacy rates or life expectancy. Abilities, in turn, are the material freedoms that individuals enjoy so as to pursue valued outcomes. The fact is that many policy frameworks do this with inputs and outputs due to their ease of measurement, but that is morally shallow. The justice-sensitive approach requires consideration of both outcomes and capabilities, which are more difficult to measure yet more ethically valuable. Equal per capita expenditures on education, to take an example, may seem equitable only when considered as the per capita distribution of inputs. However, in the event that there exists consistent learning inequalities or low retention rates, then the justice argument would crumble. A capability approach goes even further and looks at whether people are truly free to bring learning about, the answer would be yes, depending on the strength of factors beyond control like social peer pressure, family responsibilities, and language discrepancies.

The Risk of Moral Reductionism

The reduction of justice to an indicator risks moral reductionism the impoverishment of a complex, contentious value into a simplistic, quantitative vehicle. This occurs on several levels. There are four dimensions of justice, which are procedural, distributive, recognitional, and relational ontologically. Indicators often compress this into one-dimensional proxies. Epistemologically, justice is constructive and situational, whereby, indicators aspire to be objective, replicable, and comparable. Politically there is debate and bargaining over justice but in indicators they would seek closure and agreement. The standardized treatment can hide the power relations and the structural exclusions as well as the lack of voices among the marginalized groups in data collection. This uniformity has the ability of eliminating aspects of justice, which do not lend themselves to measure, e.g., the dimensions of historical redress, or cultural dignity. Interestingly, some values cannot be rationally compared with numerical scales, and the attempt to do it is likely to reflect their ethical importance in an incorrect manner.

Hybrid Approaches: Combining Quantitative Rigor with Qualitative Depth

In order to address these obstacles, numerous researchers promote hybrid modes of practice or, in other words, methods of research that include both statistical evidence and qualitative investigations, stories, and participatory proceedings. This type of structure may consist of objective statistics on inequality or health disparities, subjective measures on perceived fairness and trust, process measures of inclusivity in decision-making, individual accounts of inequity, and locally generated justice standards. It is this pluralism that enables justice to be kept track of without simplifying it. The qualitative techniques can uncover the hidden injuries, can justify those anomalies in data, and can add a moral texture to any technical information. They may contribute to the transformation of indicators to be not so much informative to the policy, but as an active challenge to power by pointing out injustices, making the underprivileged heard, and triggering institutional reform (Maurya, 2022).

The attempts to incorporate justice into the measurement of quality of life (QoL) are frustrated by a normative paradox: to measure is clarify, but also incisively divide; to render visible, but also nebulously blur. Justice cannot be reduced to a mere scale since it is a moral horizon, a horizon by reference to which everything has to be measured. The role of justice ought to be mainly to serve as a meta-norm to determine the method of indicators construction, interpretation, and to be used. It should be clear in its metrics as to whether the assessment is involved with inputs, outputs, outcomes, and capabilities or whether there is sound guard against moral reductionism. The future direction where hope exists most is in the hybrid pathways that are methodologically diverse, ethically conscious, and democratically accountable. The reason why justice cannot be measured is not due to vagueness, but rather because it is a morally expansive concept. An attempt to quantify it should always be an activity that can be criticized, revised, and discussed. Justice, in this case, is not a point of measurement destination, but the continuous task, which keeps it going.

Toward a Philosophical Framework for Ethical Social Indicators

Social indicators have infused the language of decision-making spheres in the domain of public policy, development planning, and institutional governance. However, although the sophistication of metrics has gone to a higher level, their ethical principles tend to be under-theorized. The argument of this section is that the ethically significant social indicator should be understood as according to a philosophically grounded framework that is one that views measurement as a normative practice rather than as a neutral instrument of any given administrative law. The necessity of such a frame can be illustrated by the fact when seeking to inform the policy process; indicators do the very opposite because they reproduce existing injustices through exclusion of some communities or advantage of some forms of knowledge or reducing complex morality to manageable statistics. Accordingly, the construction and implementation of indicators should have four major normative principles: transparency, reflexivity, contestability, and pluralism. All of these principles are intended to refocus measurement-as-technocratic-simplification in the direction of moral progress and democratic engagement.

Transparency, Reflexivity, Contestability, and Pluralism

The normative indicators should start with transparency, not just about the sources of the data and the methods used but also about the normative premises made. Too often, indicators present themselves as value-free or self-evident, when in fact they encode particular worldviews, definitions of well-being, and hierarchies of importance (Merry, 2011). An example of some possible normative assumptions is the Human Development Index that presumes that health, education, and income are of equal importance in human flourishing, yet again, this is a normative statement given technical-design clothing. Reflexivity demands that indicators be subject to critical self-examination. As Michael Power (1997) has argued, the culture of "audit" in governance creates mechanisms of control that can displace substantive reflection. An ethics measure should always pose the question: What is telling this measure? What does it obscure? What is being authorized or denied in terms of what kinds of lives and values? Contestability refers to the fact that there is no indicator that is irreversible or unchallengeable. In contrast to natural laws, however, social indicators are institutional constructions that are lodged in power-saturated situations. They must be open to deliberation, revision, and dissent. Amartya Sen (1993) emphasizes this in his argument for public reasoning: indicators must provoke discussion about the terms and standards of evaluation, especially among those most affected. Consequently, there is pluralism, which demands that there be more than one legitimate value system. There is no one indicator, even in a world of cultural, epistemic, and moral diversity that encompasses all that it means to live well or live justly. Ethical measurement should thus permit methodological heterodoxy, criteria sensitivity, and modesty of norms.

The Need for Epistemic Pluralism

Epistemic narrowness of social indicators is one of the most crucial ethical criticisms of the indicators. Standard metrics privilege quantitative data, expert knowledge, and Western epistemologies, while marginalizing experiential knowledge, narrative forms, and indigenous ways of knowing (de Santos, 2014; Fricker, 2007). This is not just an epistemic omission but rather an injustice as it can be called epistemic injustice that is to say people are deprived of the ability of contributing to the production of knowledge. de Santos (2014) similarly calls for cognitive justice, arguing that social evaluation systems must incorporate "epistemologies of the South," non-hegemonic knowledges rooted in historical and geographical contexts often excluded from global metric regimes. Participatory methods are key here. When they, the communities, codesign the indicators against which they will be judged," deliberative forums, participatory action research, citizen scorecards," then the process turns, not only evaluative, into emancipatory. These approaches understand the importance of having individuals with critical understanding of forms, causes, and solutions to injustice due to the fact that these people are its victims. Narrative data also plays a crucial role. The stories, testimonies, and case studies add a moral dimension to lifeless metrics, though they cannot be reduced to certian numbers. They bring not only what is going on, but how it feels, what it is, why it matters, all of which are dimensions to justice and too often obliterated by conventional measures.

Indicators as Tools of Critique, Not Just Assessment

The conventional wisdom considers indicators as monitoring and evaluation tools: to calculate performance of the institution, to follow progress, or to distribute resources. A more ambitious normative vision, however, regards them as instruments of criticism—things that can be used to unveil the shadow of injustice, to provoke a questioning awareness of the accepted ways of doing things, and to provoke active discussion of the principles on which society is organized. (Maurya, 2024). In this spirit, social indicators are akin to what Nancy Fraser (1995) calls "counterpublic discourses"—mechanisms by which marginalized groups can contest dominant frames of recognition and redistribution. As an example, the indicator pointing out racial differences in maternal mortality is not only a health indicator as well, but a diagnostic of structural racism. It invites not technocratic tinkering but normative interrogation. This transformative role of indicators aligns with what Foucault (2008) described as critique: "the art of not being governed quite so much." As designed (ethically), indicators play a more complex role than they simply serve power; they problematize power, make it contestable, and redefine what is countable.

Toward Moral Progress, Not Administrative Simplification

The question of what can be measured easily, replicated reliably, and scaled up worldwide, has too frequently been used as a design driver of indicators. This mode of orientation stresses simplicity, comparability, efficiency, which are merits in bureaucracy as well as vices in moral reasoning. The result is indicators that manage complexity by eliminating it, producing what Amartya Sen (2009) calls "informational narrowness." By contrast, a truly ethical benchmark needs to aspire to moral growth: of increasing fairness, of finding adverse views that have been marginalized, of enhancing human powers, and of fostering dignity. This requires resisting the tyranny of what Sally Engle Merry (2011) calls "governance by indicators," where the indicator becomes an end in itself, rather than a means to human flourishing. Instead, we must move toward what Sen (1993) envisions as democratic measurement: one grounded in deliberation, pluralism, and open-ended normative inquiry. The indicators under this model are not specific scorecards but ethical provocations—appeals toward reflection, reconsideration, and reimagining the metrics of a good society.

It has suggested a philosophical basis to the informal normative structure of ethical social indicators, which are rooted in the values of transparency, reflexivity, contestability, and pluralism, and dedicated to the epistemic inclusion and moral responsibility. This kind of structure lends itself to opposing a nihilistic depreciation of justice to numbers while validating the practice of measuring as the device of disenthrallment. When ethically designed, social indicators can be applied to more than gauging the development process—they can help determine moral horizons, highlight invisible injustices, and lead to the rebuilding of democracy. They are able to enable the change of words in the question by focusing on how they are performing into who they are becoming. And by doing so, they can help to bring us nearer to the sort of society where justice doesn't just measure up, but is meaningfully delivered.

Concluding Summary

Central to questioning this is a philosophical paradox at the center of answering the question, that is, how justice, in all its irreducibly normative, context-sensitive, and pluralistic sense, could be empirically measured at all? Social indicators are the pursuit of what is in the darkness in the hopes of making it light, what is qualitative in an attempt to measure the measurement, and what often is incommensurable brought to standard. One does not overcome this paradox with just a methodological trick, but with an ontological and epistemic one. In a certain way, measuring justice is also violating its nature as such as a moral ideal that cannot be reduced. And still, to give up the attempt to rank justice is to court normative insignificance when it comes to the formulation of public policy. The unmeasurable is also in large measure the unseen, and the unseen is unpracticed. In that regard, the task is not to deny quantification, but to philosophically recreate it, i.e., render it ethically transparent, epistemically diverse, and normatively self-authenticating. This concluding part of the discussion of the social indicators describes a critical-constructive philosophy on measurement in summary to cover the ethical tensions and guidelines on how justice can inform the indicators and indicators can inform justice on the quality of life. It also peeps at the coming chapter task, i.e., reframing the issue of justice as a social indicator in its own right.

Between Abstraction and Operationalization

The dangers of these efforts to measure justice are that in the quest of making justice tractable to institutions, one does what Bernard Williams (1985) mentioned as a deplorable thing, which is moral flattening: stripping something critical of its tone and intensity in the efforts to make it palatable to theory and institution. Nevertheless, abstraction is not the enemy of justice. Abstraction allows for generalization, comparability, and institutionalization—the very tools necessary for social coordination and policy application (Nussbaum, 2011). The point is not to abolish abstraction but to discipline it via critical thinking, being sure that it is also based on living realities and integral discussion. The aim of justice would not therefore be to quantify justice as such, but the conditions under which justice is realized in the form of relations and structures more or less fully. Included here is monitoring allocation of goods, opportunities and recognition, analysis of procedural fairness, and assessment of the ability of the individuals to transform material resources into decent lives.

Quantification as a Moral and Epistemic Practice

The prevailing discourse about indicators concerns them as technocratic instruments rectified neutral instruments of description that are alien to normative systems. Against this, a growing body of scholarship insists that measurement is always morally and epistemically situated (de Santos, 2014; Merry, 2011). The determination of indicator, the type of category to use, and the thresholds used are all biased decisions. Additionally, indicators are not only reflective, but rather constitutive: they focus the eye of what is perceived, what is appreciated, and what is performed. As Foucault (2008) argued, they are techniques of "governmentality," not just measuring reality but producing it in accordance with governing rationalities. In order to quantify in an ethically and epistemically answerable manner therefore demands a fundamental reconsideration of indicator implementation, development, and reading. This includes transparency in methodological assumptions; reflexivity in recognizing the limits and biases of data; epistemic pluralism, including the integration of experiential knowledge, narrative testimony, and indigenous perspectives; and democratic contestability, enabling those affected by metrics to participate in their construction and critique (Fricker, 2007; Sen, 2009). It is only after this that indicators can become devices of moral visibility instead of figuring out epistemic exclusion.

One of the major points made in this chapter has been the conflict of seeing justice as a measurable variable on the one hand, and justice as a normative system on the other. Although there are efforts in establishing direct measures of justice, e.g.,

Rule of Law Index, Perceptions of Justice Surveys, their resultant measurement tends to equate justice with reducing proxies, e.g., institutional trust or procedural compliance. This instrumentalization, although not altogether useless, threatens to reduce justice to a statistic: a figure that has lost its philosophical richness, multicultural embeddedness, and political struggle. What is even more defensible is to regard justice as a second-order evaluation criterion: not a measurement that we make, but a gathering lens in front of all of our other measurements (Maurya, 2025). A quality of life (QoL) indicator is fair in this account so long as it includes distributive justice, recognizational sensitivity to marginal identities, treats procedural inclusivity as its design feature, and incorporates emancipatory motives as opposed to simple administrative utility. The concept of justice will then become the meta-indicator of measurement itself, the morale of measure of the gauge of the moral initiative with which such a measure is validated or discredited. The critique of indicators has focused on their use in neoliberal governance: their alignment with performance management, audit cultures, and technocratic control (Espeland & Sauder, 2007; Power, 1997). However, indicators can also be used in critical and constructive ways as they can assist to diagnose injustice, bring structural violence into light, and trigger the development of moral discourse. Such an indicator of gender wage gaps does not simply describe and wait to be discussed; it becomes mobilized in a normative light and creates controversy around the idea of institutional sexism, devalued care work, and social reproduction. On the same note, clues to either educational inequality or environmental degradation may turn into moral wake-up calls to inform citizens and governments of a normative breakdown. In order to accommodate such a role, specific indicators should be placed in those institutions that are critical ones, venues of democratic debate, places of moral reasoning, and places of social struggle (Michalos & Land, 2018). They should not be accepted as any ultimate judgments, but as appeals, prompting to consider, to debate, and to review the social.

Looking Forward: Justice as a Social Measure of Quality of Life

The presence of this ending reflection previews the thematic shift into Chap. 4 where justice is not only an evaluator of indicators but offered as an indicator too, a measurable aspect of societal well-being. There are ethical opportunities to be seized in this shift, along with methodological complexities. What would it look like to come up with indicators that would measure the inequality of capabilities, under-recognition, or epistemic harms? How can measurement go beyond economic growth to include dignity, agency, and respect as well? Is it possible to come up with justice dashboards that mirror multidimensional, plural, and participatory measurements? These are questions that will be taken up in Chap. 4, based on the philosophical groundwork that this chapter is establishing and in order to construct a normatively rich theory of justice as a social indicator designed to be critical, reductive, and pluralistic, as well as ethically and politically transformational.

Measurement is not a neutral act. It is an ethical act—an act that determines the way we perceive the world, how we share resources and how we identify ourselves. Measuring justice is to assume responsibility in the terms of what and who is visible, what and how one compares, and what and when one acts. This chapter has also contended that justice should not only be the standard of our indicators but also must be the justice of our measurements. It should direct design, challenge assumptions, and excite the uses of social indicators (Michalos & Hatch, 2020). By so doing we can go to the point of a world dominated by measurement to determine justice to one where domination is by justice to determine measurement.

References

Alkire, S., & Santos, M. E. (2010). "Acute Multidimensional Poverty: A New Index for Developing Countries." *OPHI Working Paper No. 38.*

Anderson, E. (1993). *Value in ethics and economics*. Harvard University Press.

Berlin, I. (1969). *Four essays on liberty*. Oxford University Press.

Berlin, I. (1998). *The crooked timber of humanity*. Princeton University Press.

Bourdieu, P. (1984). *Distinction: A social critique of the judgement of taste*. Harvard University Press.

Cartwright, N. (2007). *Hunting causes and using them: Approaches in philosophy and economics*. Cambridge University Press.

Cartwright, N., & Montuschi, E. (Eds.). (2014). *Philosophy of social science: A new introduction*. Oxford University Press.

Cartwright, N., & Morgan, M. S. (Eds.). (1999). *The philosophy of economics: Models and matters of fact*. Oxford University Press.

Collins, P. H. (2000). *Black feminist thought*. Routledge.

Crenshaw, K. (1989). Demarginalizing the intersection of race and sex. *University of Chicago Legal Forum*, 139–167.

Crisp, R. (2013). Well-Being. In E. N. Zalta (Ed.), *The Stanford encyclopedia of philosophy (fall 2013 edition).*

de Santos, B. S. (2014). *Epistemologies of the south: Justice against Epistemicide*. Routledge.

Diener, E., Suh, E., Lucas, R. E., & Smith, H. L. (1999). Subjective Well-being: Three decades of Progress. *Psychological Bulletin, 125*(2), 276–302.

Engle Merry, S. (2011). Measuring the world: Indicators, human rights, and global governance. *Current Anthropology, 52*(S3), S83–S95.

Espeland, W. N., & Sauder, M. (2007). Rankings and reactivity: How public measures recreate social worlds. *American Journal of Sociology, 113*(1), 1–40.

Foucault, M. (1977). *Discipline and punish: The birth of the prison*. Pantheon.

Foucault, M. (2008). *The birth of biopolitics: Lectures at the Collège de France, 1978–1979*. Palgrave Macmillan.

Fraser, N. (1995). From redistribution to recognition? Dilemmas of justice in a 'post-socialist' age. *New Left Review, 212*, 68–93.

Fraser, N. (2003). *Justice interruptus: Critical reflections on the "Postsocialist" condition*. Routledge.

Fricker, M. (2007). *Epistemic injustice: Power and the ethics of knowing*. Oxford University Press.

Fukuda-Parr, S., & McNeill, D. (2019). Knowledge and politics in setting and measuring the SDGs: Introduction to special issue. *Global Policy, 10*(1), 5–15.

Fukuda-Parr, S., & Yamin, A. E. (2017). The Power of numbers: A critical review of millennium development goal targets for human development and human rights. *Journal of Human Development and Capabilities, 18*(1), 1–21.
Griffin, J. (1986). *Well-being: Its meaning, measurement and moral importance*. Oxford University Press.
Hacking, I. (1990). *The taming of chance*. Cambridge University Press.
Haybron, D. M. (2008). *The pursuit of unhappiness: The elusive psychology of Well-being*. Oxford University Press.
Honneth, A. (1995). *The struggle for recognition*. MIT Press.
Kahneman, D., & Krueger, A. B. (2006). Developments in the measurement of subjective Well-being. *Journal of Economic Perspectives, 20*(1), 3–24.
Klugman, J., Rodríguez, F., & Choi, H. J. (2011). The HDI 2010: New controversies, old critiques. *Journal of Economic Inequality, 9*, 249–288.
Kuznets, S. (1934). *National Income, 1929–1932*. U.S. Department of Commerce.
Layard, R. (2005). *Happiness: Lessons from a new science*. Penguin.
Maurya, S. K. (2020). A reply to Louis P. Pojman's article "the case against affirmative action.". *Conatus—Journal of Philosophy, 5*(2), 87–113.
Maurya, S. K. (2021). The concept of justice in reference with philosophies of Plato and Aristotle: A critical study. *Journal of Liberty and International Affairs, 7*(3), 250–266. https://doi.org/10.47305/JLIA21370250m
Maurya, S. K. (2022). On just, justice and distributive justice: A critical and comparative discourse. *Journal of Liberty and International Affairs, 8*(2), 240–254. https://doi.org/10.47305/JLIA2282240m
Maurya, S. K. (2024). African philosophies of justice and equity: A contemporary discourse. *African Journal of Religion, Philosophy and Culture, 5*(2), 61–78. https://doi.org/10.31920/2634-7644/2024/v5n2a4
Maurya, S. K. (2025). Restorative justice and karmic justice: Ubuntu and Vedanta in dialogue. *African Journal of Religion, Philosophy and Culture, 6*(2).
Merry, S. E. (2011). Measuring the world: Indicators, human rights, and global governance. *Current Anthropology, 52*(S3), S83–S95.
Michalos, A. C., & Hatch, P. M. (2020). Good societies, financial inequality and secrecy, and a good life: From Aristotle to Piketty. *Applied Research in Quality of Life, 15*(3), 1005–1054. https://doi.org/10.1007/s11482-019-09717-0
Michalos, A. C., & Land, K. C. (2018). Replies to our commentators. *Social Indicators Research, 135*(3), 1057–1078. https://doi.org/10.1007/s11205-017-1550-3
Mignolo, W. D. (2011). *The darker side of Western modernity: Global futures, Decolonial options*. Duke University Press.
Mill, J. S. (1861). *Utilitarianism*. Parker, Son, and Bourn.
Noll, H. (2002). *Social indicators and quality of life research: Background, achievements and current trends*. Sociological Institute (ZUMA).
Nussbaum, M. (2000). *Women and human development: The capabilities approach*. Cambridge University Press.
Nussbaum, M. (2006). *Frontiers of justice: Disability, nationality, species membership*. Harvard University Press.
Nussbaum, M. (2011). *Creating capabilities: The human development approach*. Harvard University Press.
OECD. (2011). *How's life? Measuring Well-being*. OECD Publishing.
Parfit, D. (1984). *Reasons and persons*. Oxford University Press.
Power, M. (1997). *The audit society: Rituals of verification*. Oxford University Press.
Rawls, J. (1971). *A Theory of Justice*. Harvard University Press.
Robeyns, I. (2005). The capability approach: A theoretical survey. *Journal of Human Development, 6*(1), 93–117.
Scanlon, T. M. (1998). *What we owe to each other*. Harvard University Press.

Searle, J. R. (1995). *The construction of social reality*. Free Press.
Sen, A. (1985). *Commodities and capabilities*. Oxford University Press.
Sen, A. (1992). *Inequality reexamined.* Harvard University Press.
Sen, A. (1993). Capability and Well-being. In *The quality of life* (pp. 30–53). Oxford University Press.
Sen, A. (1999). *Development as freedom.* Oxford University Press.
Sen, A. (2009). *The idea of justice*. Harvard University Press.
Spivak, G. C. (1988). Can the subaltern speak? In C. Nelson & L. Grossberg (Eds.), *Marxism and the interpretation of culture* (pp. 271–313). University of Illinois Press.
Talberth, J., Cobb, C., & Slattery, N. (2007). *The genuine Progress indicator 2006: A tool for sustainable development.* Redefining Progress.
UNDP. (2020). *Human development report 2020: The next frontier—Human development and the Anthropocene*. United Nations Development Programme.
Ura, K., Alkire, S., Zangmo, T., & Wangdi, K. (2012). *An extensive analysis of GNH index.* Centre for Bhutan Studies.
Williams, B. (1985). *Ethics and the limits of philosophy*. Harvard University Press.

Chapter 4
Justice as a Social Indicator

Introduction

It is needless to mention that social indicators have become essential instruments in the modern debate on the topics of public policy and societal development, allowing us to assess and contrast the quality of life of various populations. In its general understanding, a social indicator refers to a quantitative index that describes elements of societal well-being, such as, health, education, income distribution, and political involvement (Land, 2001). What is measured by these indicators does not only influence governmental and institutional decision-making but also demonstrates the normative values that a society aspires to. They are not, consequently, value-neutral; instead, they are permeated with philosophical assumptions concerning what a good society is. Traditionally, social indicators have been concerned with material and economic aspects of life, e.g., GDP per capita or unemployment rate, but over time they have begun to focus on more qualitative aspects of life such as happiness (Helliwell et al., 2020), life satisfaction (Diener et al., 1999), and capabilities (Sen, 1993). It is, however, a serious epistemic and moral lacuna that most global and national quality-of-life measures do not consider justice, especially as an independent, operationalized variable. The argument presented in this chapter, thus, concerns not only the fact that justice is a moral or political ideal but that justice is a quantifiable and act-able aspect of societal well-being that warrants consideration as a fundamental social indicator.

It is not just an oversight that justice has been left out of most statistical schemes; it indicates a more fundamental philosophical and political uneasiness. Justice is multiple, conflicting, and contextual, but so are most of the current indicators, such as subjective well-being and human freedom. The distinctive feature of justice is its normative centrality: not only is justice the constitutional system of democratic societies, but it is also the standard according to which democratic societies justify

S. K. Maurya, *Exploring Justice as a Social Indicator of Life*, Social Indicators Research Series 92, https://doi.org/10.1007/978-3-032-10812-8_4

their policies (Rawls, 1971; Sen, 2009). Failing to include justice in our assessment of societal progress is, a failure to recognize the foundation of democratic legitimacy.

Moreover, justice connects with all existing areas of social indicators. For example, health inequalities are not only a matter of biology or access but a systemic injustice issue that is bounded with race, caste, gender, and class (Marmot, 2005). Educational inequality represents a failure of justice in distribution of opportunities as well as a statistical gap (Nussbaum, 2011). Even economic measures like income inequality cannot measure up the procedural and recognitional aspects of justice, how decisions are taken, whose voices are taken into consideration and which identities are honored (Fraser, 2008). Therefore, the approach of handling justice as a cross-cutting theme without providing it with an indicator status is methodologically unsound and ethically unacceptable. This chapter picks up the immediately theoretical foundation of Chaps. 1 and 2, in which justice was determined as a philosophical mandate and a conceivable empirical abstraction. Whereas Chap. 1 introduced justice as a critical prism through which the quality of life must be interpretation, Chap. 2 followed the development of justice through classical Greek philosophy to its modern iteration in capability theory. The present chapter brings the perspective out of the theoretical and into the operationalized, it is no longer just what justice is, but how it can be measured, and more importantly, why it needs to be measured.

Further, this discussion critically responds to the debates presented in Chap. 3 concerning current measures of quality of life. Although Chap. 3 showed the advantages and shortcomings of using indicators like HDI, Gini coefficient, and subjective well-being indices, this chapter questions the fact that those indicators fail to capture normative issues. Is it possible to regard a nation as socially fair when it is the lair of racial profiling, caste-based exclusion, or gendered violence despite its high GDP and life expectancy? The response, this chapter argues, is no, and in that languages lies the case of justice as a stand-alone, measurable social indicator. The demand of justice as a quantifiable aspect is not unprecedented empirically. Already, organizations such as the World Justice Project have created justice indices that are determined by the state of the rule of law, access to civil justice, and limits on government power (World Justice Project, 2023). Yet, they are marginal to the quality-of-life reporting mainstream, usually sequestered in legal or governance ghettos. The argument presented in this chapter is that those measures need to be embedded into central well-being dashboards not as an add-on but as indicators of the moral health of a society. Overall, this chapter triggers a paradigmatic cast of discourse in terms of social indicators. It argues that not only does justice need to be rescued out of abstraction and planted back into empirical judgment as a matter of democratic pride, but as a matter of sound policy. By so doing, it intends to form the foundation of a multidimensional justice indicator, a justice indicator that is philosophically valid, culturally responsive, and empirically supported.

Historical and Philosophical Context

The problem of justice has held a seminal position in both Western and non-Western philosophical thought over the last 2000 years. But in spite of this central concern in moral and political philosophy, the subject of justice has been noticeably missing in the realm of empirical social measurement. This seeming contradiction in which justice is idealized as one of the highest of moral values, yet is seldom put into statistical operation as a social measure, represents a deep division between the logic of philosophical thought and the logic of quantitative social research. To reintroduce justice into modern schemes of social evaluation, it is essential to start with the conceptual lineage of justice, as developed by philosophers since Plato up to Nussbaum, and to evaluate critically the conceptual incompatibilities between the moral and the statistical sense of justice.

Justice in Classical Philosophy: Seeking Order and Harmony

The metaphysical and hierarchical nature of Plato justice most famously set forth in *The Republic*. For Plato, justice exists when "each part of the soul and each class of society performs its appropriate function". It is inner harmony, social order, and not a measure of results. The concept of justice is closely related to functional specialization than to distributive equality, a view deeply rooted in his belief in a tripartite soul and tripartite society. Though the concept of justice introduced by Plato forms a cornerstone of normative theory, it could hardly contribute to the building of justice as a social indicator, namely because it is aesthetic and idealistic instead of being procedural and empirical.

In contrast, Aristotle starts to establish the foundations of empirical thought on justice. In *Nicomachean Ethics*, he distinguishes between distributive justice, which concerns the fair allocation of resources, and corrective justice, which pertains to the rectification of wrongs (Aristotle, 2009). The idea of proportional equality, of giving to each according to their merit, which Aristotle stresses, anticipates later discussions of meritocracy and social equality. Yet his framework, while richer in practical implications than Plato's, still embeds justice within a teleological view of human flourishing (eudaimonia) rather than viewing it as a stand-alone criterion for governance or policy analysis.

Modern Theories: From Morality to Measurability

Modern political philosophy, and especially the liberal tradition, is where justice starts to gain normative power, as well as depth in procedure. John Rawls' *A Theory of Justice* (1971) marks a decisive break from classical essentialism. Rawls conceptualizes justice as fairness, grounded in the two principles of equal basic liberties and fair equality of opportunity, regulated by the difference principle, which allows social and economic inequalities only if they benefit the least advantaged (Rawls, 1971). Not only does Rawls moralize institutional design, but he also injects a quasi-mathematical logic into the discussion of justice by instruments such as the original position and veil of ignorance. It is this procedural rigor that brings justice a step closer to be formalized, although not yet quantified, in social assessment.

Nevertheless, the use of the ideal theory by Rawls has been criticized as being out of touch with actual injustices in the world. Amartya Sen's The Idea of Justice (2009) offers a counterpoint through his comparative, nonideal approach, emphasizing public reasoning and actual realizations over hypothetical contracts. Sen refutes the institutionalism of Rawls in favor of capabilities and freedoms, thus connecting justice to well-being in a manner that makes it open to empirical investigation. According to Sen, justice is about the expansion of people's capabilities to live the kind of life they have reason to value (Sen, 1993, 2009). His influence is visible in the Human Development Index (HDI), which attempts to move beyond GDP by including life expectancy, education, and per capita income. Martha Nussbaum extends Sen's capability approach with a clearly defined list of central human capabilities, asserting that any society that fails to secure these is manifestly unjust (Nussbaum, 2011). Her model is a veiled demand on a universal but culturally aware set of justice standards. In contrast to Rawls and his consideration of idealized citizens in a closed society, Nussbaum and Sen are taking the justice discourse into the area of international development, social indicators, and human rights a step that becomes the philosophical foundation of the main argument in this chapter.

Moral Justice Versus Statistical/Social Justice

One obstacle to the embrace of justice as a social indicator is the false contrast between moral justice and statistical/social justice. Moral justice is traditionally considered a qualitative domain, concerned with fairness, ethics, and virtue, while statistical justice is viewed as inherently reductionist, prone to abstraction and loss of nuance (Maurya, 2024). This binary is unhelpful but also epistemically regressive in that it sustains a separation that inhibits the possibility of cross-pollination between ethics and empirical research. Upon further examination, most of the existing indicators already have moral values coded within them, even if only implicitly. Consider, e.g., the Gini coefficient that is said to gauge income inequality yet it is merely an indicator of how society is willing to put up with distributive injustice. Similarly, the World Happiness Report ranks nations by subjective well-being, which reflects deep-seated assumptions about what constitutes a good life (Helliwell et al., 2020). In this way, the distinction between moral justice and statistical justice is an illusion, the heritage of disciplinary compartments, not the dictate of philosophy. The question, then, is not whether justice is measurable, but how without diminishing its moral gravity, to make it measurable. Measuring justice should not be reductionist but multidimensional. It must capture not just distributive outcomes but also procedural justice (fairness in decision-making) and recognitional justice (respect for diverse identities), dimensions that scholars such as Nancy Fraser (2008) and Iris Marion Young (1990) have emphasized as crucial to any meaningful justice framework.

Influence on Quality-of-Life Paradigms and Social Indicators

Though philosophical theories of justice have long been reserved within the normative sphere, their mark upon the quality of life (QoL) paradigms is undeniable. The capability approach by Sen has radically transformed the way development is evaluated by economists and policy-makers. The UNDP's Human Development Reports explicitly acknowledge Sen's work as foundational in moving beyond income-centric metrics (UNDP, 1990, 2020). Similarly, the OECD Better Life Index incorporates civic engagement or work–life balance as some of its dimensions, criteria that imply more underlying ethical commitment to equity and freedom.

However, with these developments, the majority of quality of life (QoL) models do not go as far as to include justice itself as an indicator. They measure its symptoms (inequality, exclusion, corruption) but not the conceptual center. It is comparable to quantifying the health of the population by illness rates and neglecting systemic factors such as clean air or nondiscriminatory access to care. The way to actually make justice a part of social science is the route shown by Sen and Nussbaum, justice should not be considered as primarily an ideal to be aspired toward but a structural state whose presence or absence can and should be recorded. Further, philosophical theories of justice promise more than moral justification; they promise analytical infrastructure to construct empirical models. Policy simulations can be directed by Rawlsian principles of fairness, and survey tools and rubrics can be informed by the capabilities of Nussbaum. The linking of philosophy and measurement is not just feasible, but needed. Without it, we risk mistaking statistical adequacy for ethical adequacy, a danger that becomes particularly acute in neoliberal contexts where metrics often displace meaning (Merry, 2011).

What Makes a Good Social Indicator?

The value of social indicators has been found in making visible, actionable, and accountable in policy circles, complex aspects of human well-being. However, what constitutes a good social indicator is highly disputed in both theory and practice. Traditional requirements include objectivity, measurability, policy relevance, cultural sensitivity, and temporal consistency (Land, 2001; Noll, 2002). Although such criteria offer a basis of analysis, they also expose a normative bias and disciplinary assumptions that tend to fetishize more contentious and multifaceted constructs such as justice. This part challenges the attributes of a good social indicator, questions how the mainstream indicators measure up to (or fall short of) these attributes, and demonstrates justice as a disruptor and as an inevitable next step in the indicator paradigm.

Objectivity: The Mirage of Neutrality

It is common to idealize objectivity as the ideal of good indicators, the gold standard. It implies that indicators should be detached from ideological positions and based on replicable, quantitative data (Noll, 2002). However, as many scholars have pointed out, no social indicator is ideologically neutral; they are always shaped by value judgments about what counts as "good" or "desirable" in society (Merry, 2011; Sen, 1993). The Human Development Index (HDI), for instance, combines life expectancy, education, and income into a single composite score. While widely celebrated, it embodies implicit normative claims about what constitutes development, privileging formal education over indigenous knowledge systems, or income over social capital (UNDP, 2020).

The myth of objectivity is productively challenged by justice. It compels us to address the moral aspects that underlie social indicators instead of seeking refuge behind technocratic priests. A justice indicator, by necessity, involves subjective perceptions (e.g., fairness, dignity), institutional structures (e.g., rule of law), and cultural contexts (e.g., caste, race, or gender norms), elements that resist simplification but offer deeper epistemological insight into social realities. The clamor of objectivity should not be made a tool of keeping out the morally relevant.

Measurability: The Limits of Quantification

Measurability is yet another paramount criterion: the assumption that indicators should be subject to statistical treatment, making it possible to compare over time and space. Measurement tools such as Gini coefficient (a measure of inequality of income) are popular due to their simplicity in mathematics and their universality. However, measurability can also become a straightjacket, favoring what is easily counted over what is ethically meaningful (Espeland & Stevens, 2008).

Justice interferes with this rationality by showing the boundaries of quantification. Is it sensible to quantify the anguish of caste-based indignities, the trauma of racial profiling, or the indignity of unequal access to the law? These are questions that cannot be answered with neat numerical values, but which must be asked in order to determine the health of society. This does not mean justice is unmeasurable, but rather that it requires a multimethod approach, combining quantitative tools (like access to legal aid or representation in decision-making bodies) with qualitative inputs (like testimonial narratives or lived experiences) (Fraser, 2008; Sen, 2009). Measurability, that is, should not patrol conceptual precincts but enlarge its methodological tool box.

Policy Relevance: Technocracy Versus Transformative Potential

The third criterion is policy relevance, the notion that indicators should be directly useful in decision-making. Indicators like the Multidimensional Poverty Index (MPI) or the Global Peace Index (GPI) are popular because they translate social phenomena into policy levers: a rise in poverty or conflict becomes a call to action (Alkire & Santos, 2010; IEP (Institute for Economics and Peace), 2023). However, these indicators tend to validate the status quo in that they look at outcomes without questioning the power structures that influence that outcome. Justice offers a more transformative potential for policy relevance. The justice indicator could serve not merely as a diagnostic but also as a normative standard against which every other policy could be evaluated. To provide some examples, where an improvement in GDP corresponds with a strengthening of social exclusion or a breach in procedural fairness, a justice indicator would show this as a step backward instead of a positive achievement by a government policy. This would add a moral sieve to policy analysis that is absent in present indicators. Moreover, justice-based indicators can support intersectional policy-making, identifying how multiple forms of disadvantage interact—such as gender, race, class, and disability—to produce complex forms of injustice (Crenshaw, 1991; Nussbaum, 2011). This is especially acute in multicultural societies such as Indian or South African, where a blanket policy frequently cannot cope with deeply rooted systemic disparities.

Cultural Sensitivity: Navigating Universality and Pluralism

Ideally, the most desirable social indicators are those that are responsive to cultural settings, at the same time maintaining international comparability. This balance is notoriously difficult. The HDI, for example, has been critiqued for applying Western-centric notions of development globally. Even subjective well-being indicators, while claiming universality, often mask cultural biases in how emotions and life satisfaction are expressed (Diener et al., 1999). Justice, more than most indicators, demands a pluralistic framework. What is considered just in one legal or cultural tradition is not necessarily seen as such in another one. But this does not imply an argument against measurement, it implies an argument for contextualized measurement. Justice indicators can be tailored to account for local norms, historical grievances, and sociopolitical structures, while still adhering to basic global principles such as nondiscrimination, equity, and human dignity (Rawls, 1971; Sen, 2009). For example, the access to justice in tribal regions, which may necessitate various criteria than in metropolitan cities; gender justice in societies that are patriarchal should concentrate not just on legal equality, but on cultural change. The validity of justice as a social indicator, therefore, is strengthened and not weakened by cultural sensitivity.

Such indicators as the MPI or Gini coefficient enable policy-makers to monitor poverty or inequality trends over decades. Nonetheless, most indicators provide point-in-time pictures, which do not reflect the historical injustices or intergenerational impacts. Justice, in contrast, inherently incorporates temporal depth. It cares not only about present distributions but historic redress and future equity as well. As an illustration, affirmative action programs are frequently defended not just based on current inequalities but on hundreds of years of discrimination. An effective justice indicator would account for such temporal asymmetries, offering a more comprehensive ethical timeline than traditional measures allow (Fraser, 2008; Young, 1990). Moreover, justice may aid in judging readily efficient policies that may turn detrimental in the long run, thus introducing a level of moral inspection to temporal assessments. Justice not only fits but also challenges the existing paradigm of social indicators. It can, on the one hand, meet the essence criteria once adequately defined and measured: it is policy-relevant, culture-sensitive, time-profound, and, with the help of imaginative methodologies, measurable. Conversely, it questions reductionism, myths of objectivity, and technocratic neutrality that have been progressive in indicators development. Justice-based approach demands a reconceptualization of indicators as a moral, rather than a purely measuring device. It demands that we expand our understanding of what counts as knowledge, whose experiences matter, and how power is embedded in data (Merry, 2011). Consequently, justice is not a peripheral addition, a refinement; it is a paradigm change in the way we entertain, assess, and manage the society.

Conceptualizing Justice as a Social Indicator

The claim that justice must act as a social signal is not merely attractive in a normative sense, but it is also analytically compulsory. Justice is the foundation of practically all social policy aims; fair access to health care, fair legal systems, fair access to education, and so on but justice as a concept is not exploited in the development of national or international social indicators. That gap cannot be simply attributed to oversight; it somehow represents a more fundamental uneasiness with the multidimensionality of justice, its normative complexity, and its supposed immeasurability. But it is ethically unacceptable, as well as intellectually slothful, to formal indicators to exclude justice on the ground that it cannot be simplified. This part will conceptualize justice as a quantifiable social indicator by functioning its fundamental dimensions, suggesting a normative conceptualization, and discussing the epistemological and moral dilemmas inherent in its use.

The Multidimensional Nature of Justice: Beyond Redistribution

The modern conceptions of justice emphasize that justice is not a singular notion but a clustering of interlocking issues. A meaningful conceptualization must include at least four interrelated dimensions: distributive, procedural, recognitional, and restorative justice (Fraser, 2008; Young, 1990).

Distributive Justice

It is the most widely known type, which deals with equal distribution of resources and opportunities. It is the basis of such measures as the Gini coefficient, income quintiles, and Multidimensional Poverty Index. However, distributive justice does not consider how the decisions are reached, which individuals or whose identity is affirmed, and how past wrongs can be righted.

Procedural Justice

Procedural justice deals with fairness in decision-making especially in institutions like the court system, schools, and bureaucracies. Studies show that individuals often accept unfavorable outcomes if they perceive the process as fair (Tyler, 2006). Procedural justice is thus crucial for democratic legitimacy and institutional trust and should be assessed through indicators like transparency, participation, and impartial adjudication (Rawls, 1971; Sen, 2009).

Recognitional Justice

This dimension, brought to the forefront by scholars such as Nancy Fraser and Axel Honneth, refers to the respect and inclusion of cultural identities, genders, abilities, and sexualities (Fraser, 2008; Honneth, 1995). Recognitional justice deals with symbolic injuries, like misrepresentation, cultural domination, or erasure, which cannot be measured in material terms but are equally harmful to human dignity.

Restorative Justice

Restorative justice emphasizes repair and reconciliation rather than punishment. Though it is frequently limited to the circle of criminal justice, it has wider applications to societies emerging out of conflict, colonialism, or entrenched discrimination. Measures here could include reparations, truth commissions, or institutional reforms (Braithwaite, 2001; Gavrielides, 2007). Collectively, the four dimensions constitute the pillars of a comprehensive justice indicator. The omission of any of them leaves a biased and potentially distorted impression of social reality.

A Conceptual Framework for Justice Indicators

In order to incorporate justice sensibly into social indicator systems, we need to leave theory behind and work toward operationalization. This will involve developing a multilayered structure integrating structural, procedural, and outcome-based indicators.

Structural Indicators

These reflect the legal and institutional framework supporting justice. Examples include:

- Existence of antidiscrimination laws
- Access to legal representation and public defenders
- Institutional independence (judiciary, police)

Process Indicators

These assess the quality of procedures within institutions. Examples include:

- Percentage of population participating in public consultations
- Representation of marginalized groups in policy-making
- Timeliness and fairness of judicial proceedings

Outcome Indicators

These measure actual experiences and perceptions. Examples include:

- Survey-based perceived fairness of government institutions
- Rates of discriminatory practices (e.g., police profiling, workplace bias)
- Disparities in education, health care, and employment outcomes

Such a model resonates with the UN OHCHR's tripartite typology of structure-process-outcome indicators, originally developed for human rights monitoring (OHCHR, 2012). The peculiar feature of justice indicators, however, is their normative aspiration: they do not describe the world as it is; they measure how fair it is.

Normative Challenges: Justice to Whose, of Whom, and on What Grounds?

The deepest barrier to the development of justice indicators is their normative confusion. Justice, unlike GDP or literacy, is inherently contested. Whose ideal of justice must be formalized in the indicators? Do we favor liberal-individualist paradigms, communitarianism ethics, or postcolonial theories? It is not a technical question but a political question.

Whose Justice?

Western liberal traditions emphasize fairness and procedural rights (Rawls, 1971), but non-Western traditions may prioritize community harmony, reparative customs, or spiritual balance. For example, Ubuntu in Southern Africa promotes a relational concept of justice rooted in reconciliation and coexistence (Gade, 2012). Any universal indicator of justice runs the risk of epistemic violence when it tries to establish a single cultural system as valid worldwide.

Justice for Whom?

Justice is not equally felt even a single societal context. Intersectional theory demonstrates that women of color, disabled persons, or LGBTQ+ individuals face overlapping forms of injustice that are invisible in average-based indicators (Crenshaw, 1991). Therefore, the indicators of justice need to be broken down by identity markers, which will show the biases in the system. Aggregated averages conceal injustice; granularity reveals it.

Justice by What Criteria?

The attempt to construct quantifiable standards of justice welcomes both moral and procedural controversies. Should justice be evaluated through outcomes (equality of condition), opportunities (capabilities), or processes (deliberative fairness)? Amartya Sen (2009) argues against transcendent notions of "perfect justice" and advocates for a comparative, realization-focused approach. This perspective informs the advancement of context-based indicators that are anchored on a public rationale as opposed to technocratic formulae.

Moreover, the choice of indicators always reflects power. As Sally Engle Merry (2011) notes, global metrics often exclude local knowledge, indigenous epistemologies, and resistance narratives. Any such model that attempts to quantify justice must also be subject to democratic challenge and correction so that various communities may determine what justice entails in their own context. The very notion of justice as a social indicator requires nothing short of a redefinition of the measure as well. In contrast to the traditional indicators, which simply follow the progress of development, a justice-based model makes the society responsible toward its moral underpinnings. It questions authority, gives voice to the margins, and reveals systemic injustices. It is not its weakness, but the most powerful indication of justice. Justice is not too complicated to be measured; it is too serious not to be measured. The gap between moral theory and moral practice can be closed using a multidimensional, culturally sensitive, and normatively transparent indicator framework. In instilling the aspect of justice in our social indicator systems, we replace the technocratic rationality of governing with an ethics of transformation in our accountability and inclusion.

Operationalizing Justice: Methodological Considerations

The imperative to make justice operational as a social indicator is bound to elicit controversial issues on methodology, epistemology, and cultural relativism. In contrast to traditional indicators, like literacy rates or life expectancy, justice is normative, perception-based, and structure-sensitive. It does not yield to easy quantification, but requires empirical purchase, should it be used to inform policy and institutional change. The section will develop the thesis that justice is not immeasurable, but its operationalization needs a methodological pluralism that puts the reductionist impulse of traditional social science into question. It is through embracing quantitative and qualitative paradigms, perception-based and institutional measures, and facing the challenge of cross-cultural validity that we can build indicators of justice that matter and do not deprive justice of its normative depth.

Quantitative Versus Qualitative: False Binaries and Hybrid Approaches

Quantitative and qualitative research divide is one of the most enduring methodological fault lines in social science. Quantitative indicators, favored for their replicability, comparability, and policy relevance, dominate global indicator systems like the Human Development Index (UNDP, 2020) or the Global Peace Index (IEP (Institute for Economics and Peace), 2023). However, justice is intrinsically concerned with meanings, contexts, and moral assessments, which are not always adapted to quantification. Critics argue that quantifying justice dilutes its ethical content and privileges surface-level outcomes over structural analysis (Espeland & Stevens, 2008; Merry, 2011). But, by demanding specifically qualitative techniques, there is a danger of pushing justice out of the world of policy, where quantification is king to political legitimacy. The actual methodological problem is not to prefer numbers or narratives but to integrate them into a combined structure. Both philosophical or normative considerations and empirical evidence point toward a mixed-methods approach as the optimal methodology. For example, we could pair a survey-based Justice Perception Index with case studies of legal aid access, ethnographic reports of procedural bias, and policy audits of antidiscrimination enforcement. In doing so, we acknowledge that no single metric can capture justice, but a constellation of interlinked methods can approximate it meaningfully and responsibly (Fraser, 2008; Sen, 2009).

Measuring Perceptions: Surveys as Moral Thermometers

Perceptions matter deeply in justice. Studies consistently show that people's sense of procedural fairness, how they are treated by the police, courts, or employers, influences their trust in institutions more than the actual outcomes (Levi et al., 2009; Tyler, 2006). Thus, perception-based indicators are indispensable in operationalizing justice. Perceptions of fairness, judicial independence, and government accountability are regularly measured in surveys, such as the World Justice Project Rule of Law Index or the Afrobarometer and Eurobarometer. Yet, the perception data is commonly debunked as a mere "opinion" that is volatile and influenced by thinking bias. This criticism, while not entirely unfounded, overlooks a crucial fact: justice is experienced subjectively, and to ignore this is to dismiss lived realities as analytically irrelevant (Merry, 2011). Additionally, through rigorous design, triangulation, cognitive pre-testing, and cultural calibration, surveys can also offer systematic knowledge about how various groups encounter justice. When classified by class, caste, race, gender, or region, they reveal grain-level injustices that are hidden by average statistics. For example, a 2020 Pew Research Center study revealed a significant disparity in perceptions of the fairness of the judicial system, with a much lower percentage of African Americans expressing confidence in the system compared to the general population, highlighting racialized perceptions of injustice and its policy implications. (Pew Research Center, 2020). The perceptions are not, then, a distortion of reality, they are rather constitutive of it, in the matter of justice in particular.

Institutional Metrics: Mapping Structural Capacities

Perceptions are not enough; they should be combined with institutional indicators measuring how justice systems operate in practice. These indicators assess availability, accessibility, affordability, and quality of institutions and structures charged with provision of justice—Courts, legal assistance, police, and regulatory bodies.

Examples of institutional metrics include:

- The percentage of population covered by legal aid (low income population)
- Caseloads per judge or resolution time in courts (efficiency indicators)

- Existence and enforcement of antidiscrimination laws
- Funding of human rights commissions or public defenders

Such metrics are used by the OECD's Access to Justice framework (OECD, 2021) and the UN's Rule of Law Indicators (UNDP, 2009). Critics, however, note that these structural indicators tend to concentrate on formal equality without attention to substantive results. A nation can have laws against discrimination on the books but not enforce them; it can offer legal assistance in the cities but ignore the rural or tribal districts. Institutional indicators should be dynamic hence, involving performance audits, compliance checks, and participatory evaluations. Moreover, procedural fairness and institutional trust are not presumed on the basis of inputs. A justice system's effectiveness must be gauged not just by its existence, but by how equitably and ethically it functions (Fraser, 2008; Honneth, 1995).

The Cross-Cultural Challenge: Universal Aspirations or Moral Imperialism?

Perhaps the most complex methodological issue is cross-cultural validity. Not everyone perceives and encounters justice in a similar manner. In liberal societies, justice is often framed in terms of rights and procedures, while in many Indigenous, African, or Asian traditions, it may emphasize relational harmony, spiritual balance, or reparative obligations (Gade, 2012). The pursuit of a single measure of global justice carries the risk of epistemic violence and the silencing of the local conceptions in the favor of Western liberal conceptions. Nor is this a purely theoretical issue; global indices frequently fail to include non-Western institutions in their indicator framework. For example, traditional justice systems in Africa-based on mediation and community reconciliation, are rarely captured in UN or World Bank assessments of rule of law. The solution is not to give up on comparability, but to adopt pluralism in structure. The justice indicators should be grounded on universal moral values, such as nondiscrimination, dignity, freedom of violence, but with flexibility on how they are expressed and realized locally. This approach mirrors the "overlapping consensus" model of Rawls (1993), where different moral systems can agree on shared principles while retaining cultural specificity. Also, the codesigning of indicators with local communities, through participatory approaches guarantees legitimacy, and cultural appropriateness. This bottom-up epistemology aligns with decolonial research ethics and enhances indicator resilience in diverse settings (Chilisa, 2012; Smith, 1999). The project of making justice operational is not the naive or those driven by unrealistic idealism. It is a methodological imperative of any society, which purports to be morally legitimate and democratically upright. Although justice is not a single metric, it can be addressed in a meaningful way through multilayered indicators that integrate perception data, institutional measures, and qualitative stories. To do this we have to move beyond methodological purism, address our cultural biases, and transform what constitutes knowledge in policy science. Justice questions the epistemological elitism of technocratic indicators and demands that the people most harmed by injustice also be its most important epistemic actors. The era of increasing inequality, distrust of institutions, and democratic decline, measuring justice is no longer a luxury, rather it is a democratic imperative or necessity.

Justice has in recent times made inroads into the empirical landscape of governance, policy, and development. However, its operationalization is unequal and, in many cases, it mirrors local political histories, institutional capacities, and cultural values. Three comparative case studies include Nordic countries, India, and South Africa in this section that shows how justice has been integrated into social measurement frameworks. The cases raise the dimensions of justice in focus: procedural, distributive, recognitional, and restorative. They collectively make a strong case about the viability, usefulness, and boundaries of incorporating justice into public indicators.

The Nordic Countries Procedural Justice and the Welfare State Context

The Nordic countries (Sweden, Norway, Denmark, and Finland) are frequently referred to as the models of egalitarianism and social justice. They are characterized by their welfare states that are founded on the idea of universalism and which are designed to provide equality in access to resources, services, and political representation. This adherence to procedural justice, or the fairness of governance processes, is the main spine of their social model.

Method of Measurement

Nordic justice is typically measured indirectly using such indicators of justice as:

- High trust in public institutions
- Low corruption indices (Transparency International, 2022)
- Accessibility and responsiveness of public services (OECD, 2019)
- Public participation in governance (Christensen & Laegreid, 2007)

For instance, the Health and Medical Services Act in Sweden stipulates equality in access and patient rights, thus fairness in service delivery is a legally enshrined norm. Moreover, social scientists have used longitudinal surveys to assess procedural fairness in the tax system, finding that even high-income citizens tolerate steep taxation if processes are seen as transparent and redistributive (Rothstein, 2005).

The outcomes are striking. Nordic countries rank among the highest in:

- Social mobility
- Public satisfaction with government

- Well-being indexes (UNDP, 2020)

This is attributed not just to income redistribution but to the perception that institutions treat citizens fairly and equally, regardless of status (Tyler, 2006). Procedural justice here is both the means and the end.

Limitations

However, the Nordic model is not immune to critique. Immigrants and ethnic minorities often report lower trust and fairness in interactions with institutions, revealing a recognitional justice gap. In addition, universal welfare has the propensity to conceal the different treatment of justice along race and gender. Thus, even within exemplary systems, justice requires constant recalibration.

India: Affirmative Action, Caste Equity, and Legal Justice Context

India is a tricky case of an unjust system that has been historically built over centuries around the caste system, gender inequity, and religious marginalization. The Indian Constitution attempts to counteract this through a range of affirmative action policies—reservations in education, jobs, and politics for Scheduled Castes (SCs), Scheduled Tribes (STs), and Other Backward Classes (OBCs).

Method of Measurement

Justice here is approached through distributive and legal lenses. Indicators include:

- Reservation in jobs and admissions in universities in the public sector
- Budget allocations to Scheduled Castes Sub-Plan (SCSP)
- Access to justice (e.g., cases filed under the Scheduled Castes and Scheduled Tribes (Prevention of Atrocities) Act)
- Representation in political offices

Additionally, the National Crime Records Bureau (NCRB) tracks caste-based crimes, while the National Sample Survey Office (NSSO) conducts household surveys disaggregated by caste. Those are implicit tools that gauge justice by determining whether the redistributive tools diminish historical inequalities.

Affirmative action has produced some tangible benefits:

- Increased SC/ST enrollment in higher education (Deshpande, 2013)
- Political representation in local bodies (Pande, 2003)
- Constitutionalization of the caste injustice, which is normative outside of policy

However, the realization gap remains substantial. Discrimination in employment, housing, and health care persists, often in covert or systemic forms (Thorat & Newman, 2012). Institutional apathy, fear of retaliation, and stigmatization mean that legal justice mechanisms are underused.

According to the critics, justice in India is being measured in terms of quotas instead of changing lives. Moreover, by focusing narrowly on caste, the system often fails to address intersectional injustices based on gender, disability, or religion (Guru, 2000). Also, court delays and judicial backlogs water down the concept of procedural justice, especially to the marginalized groups. In this way, even though India is realizing justice in a very explicit manner, its indicator systems tend to fall short in measuring its more structural and cultural aspects.

South Africa: Postapartheid Justice and the Politics of Repair Context

The end of apartheid and the establishment of democracy in South Africa was precisely formulated as a restorative justice project. The Truth and Reconciliation Commission (TRC), led by Archbishop Desmond Tutu, became a global exemplar of how nations attempt to measure and administer justice after systemic violence.

Method of Measurement

Justice in postapartheid South Africa has been measured through:

- Number of TRC hearings and reparations issued
- Equity in land redistribution and restitution programs
- Employment Equity Index (EEI) and Broad-Based Black Economic Empowerment (B-BBEE) scores
- Surveys on social cohesion and trust in public institutions (HSRC (Human Sciences Research Council), 2020)

The Justice, Crime Prevention, and Security (JCPS) Cluster of the government also tracks legal reforms, access to justice, and police accountability. The TRC helped the country to heal itself and left a record of atrocities to the public. Symbolic justice was prioritized, and reparations, though limited, were provided. The Employment Equity Act (1998) and the Broad-Based Black Economic Empowerment Act (2003), i.e., B-BBEE Act (2003) have tried to materialize justice in the economy by correcting historic imbalances. Moreover, South Africa's constitution is one of the most progressive in the world, explicitly stating the right to human dignity, equality, and justice (Republic of South Africa, 1996).

Despite these initiatives, structural inequalities remain stark:

- The Gini coefficient is one of the highest globally (World Bank, 2022)
- Land reform has been slow and contentious

- There is a reduced trust in institutions especially by the young black South Africans

Justice in this case, though rhetorically effective, has not been easy to realize in life. The TRC, while globally praised, is critiqued for prioritizing reconciliation over accountability (Mamdani, 2002). The promise of restorative justice will not be full without deeper economic change.

Comparative Reflections: Patterns and Pitfalls

Across these three cases, some patterns emerge:

1. Justice is already being measured, but often indirectly. Justice has become a measurement issue whether it is by trust surveys in Scandinavia, or reservation statistics in India or in South Africa reconciliation. But it is hardly ever brought together into a unified indicator system.
2. Context shapes the dominant justice dimension. Procedural justice is the norm in the Nordic countries; distributive justice in India; restorative justice in South Africa. This asserts the fact that justice indicators cannot be universal in nature but rather context-sensitive.
3. Structural transformation lags behind normative commitment. All three states articulate justice as a moral imperative. But they are having trouble actually achieving it in reality, particularly with regard to intersectionality, systemic change, and long-term institutional performance.
4. Justice indicators reveal power asymmetries. Measurement is political. What gets measured, how it is interpreted, and who controls the data reflect underlying power dynamics (Merry, 2011). Justice indicators have to be democratically responsible and epistemically inclusive.

The international case studies highlight that justice is quantifiable as well as a battleground. Justice indicators are not a utopian idea: they already exist, although they are frequently fragmented, implicit, or on the weak side of the theorization. So as to realize the democratic promise of justice we have to render these indicators self-conscious, coherent, and critically aware. By studying systems as varied as the Nordic welfare states, India's affirmative action model, and South Africa's restorative apparatus, we learn not only about justice's possibilities but also its limitations. It is not simply a question of measuring justice but of questioning incessantly the systems that make justice possible or impossible.

Critiques and Limitations of Justice as a Social Indicator

Although the very desire to quantify justice as a social indicator can be viewed as a noble attempt at achieving morally sound governing and responsibility, it is both epistemologically non-neutral and politically controversial. In contrast to other indicators like GDP or life expectancy, which, although they too are controversial, are based on measurable proxies, justice comes into the picture as a normative, culturally mediated, and usually disputed value. Four main issues that are subject to critical analysis in this section are the subjectivity of perceptions of justice, the fact that measures of justice have been politicized, the universalism versus cultural relativism dilemma, and the ethical question of quantification as such.

The Subjectivity and Variability of Justice Perceptions

Critiques of justice indicators is rooted in their subjectivity. Justice, unlike literacy or income, is deeply tied to perceived fairness, which varies across individuals, communities, and cultures (Tyler, 2006). What appears just to one group of people may be perceived to be unjust to another. For instance, affirmative action policies that promote redistributive justice for historically marginalized groups may simultaneously be perceived as unjust by those who feel excluded (Sowell, 2004). By focusing on perception, surveys like those from the World Justice Project have brought lived experiences of injustice into sharper focus. Yet, these perceptions are notoriously unstable, influenced by media narratives, individual biases, and recent events (Merry, 2011). Moreover, the answers could represent an ideological congruity rather than reality of institutional performance. In that regard, the gap in justice quantified might rely more on emotional response than system malfunction. This instability threatens to compromise the usability of justice indicators in long-term policy formulation. To the extent that public perception is fluid, how can it provide a solid foundation for institutional benchmarking?, Or do we then pose the question: Ought perceptions to be corrected which are at variance with legal or institutional data? These tensions inform the epistemic uncertainty in which justice indicators need to maneuver.

Risk of Politicization in Justice Metrics

Justice indicators are inescapably political in contrast with technical indicators like inflation rates. This is because they border on issues of who receives what, how, and why, thus drawing the interests of the ruling regimes, bureaucratic agencies, and civil society into question. When governments selectively deploy justice indicators, there is a risk of symbolic politics, using metrics to signal virtue without substantive reform (Merry, 2016). For instance, authoritarian regimes may showcase justice indicators that emphasize legal order and crime reduction while suppressing indicators of procedural fairness or minority rights (Huq & Ginsburg, 2018). In even the democratic settings, justice measures run the risk of turning into policy-justification tools as opposed to being actual reform instruments. As Espeland and Stevens (2008) warn, quantification often confers "aura of objectivity," giving ideological decisions a veneer of neutrality. Still more consequences of this politicization are indicator capture, where measures are moved around to show signs of improvement without any real structural transformation. For example, increasing legal aid spending may appear as justice expansion on paper, even if accessibility barriers, such as language, geography, or corruption, remain untouched (Sen, 2009). In this way, justice cannot be separated or extracted or isolated or removed or divested of power, and any measure that presents itself as a measure of justice must also contend with how measures themselves can be colonized by the interests of power.

Universalism Versus Cultural Relativism: Whose Justice?

The second line of criticism questions, whether justice indicators can be universally applied or must account for cultural variation, an essential philosophical debate. While liberal political philosophy, especially in the Rawlsian and Senian traditions, attempts to ground justice in universally applicable norms like fairness, freedom, and equity (Maurya, 2021), anthropologists and postcolonial scholars caution against exporting such frameworks into culturally diverse contexts. Most non-Western cultures place justice within the context of relationships and communities rather than individual rights. The concept of Ubuntu in Southern Africa, or Dharma in Indian philosophy, reflects justice not as an abstract principle but as context-sensitive harmony (Gade, 2012). As the world meters become dominated by liberal-legalistic concepts of justice, there is a threat of epistemic imperialism: the imposition of a strongly limited concept of the world in the name of neutrality. This leads to an urgent methodological and ethical dilemma: Is there a way to have a global justice indicator without leveling the particularities of the cultures? Or should indicators be radically localized, hence forfeiting international comparability? The quest to find universal metrics of justice is therefore based on a paradox; what makes indicators internationally valid, typically renders them nationally invalid or even unjust.

Ethical Critique: Should Everything Be Quantified?

The last, and possibly the most philosophically challenging, objection is a challenge to the very assumption of measuring justice. Justice, some argue, is not a thing to be measured but a moral horizon that should guide action and critique, not institutional performance scores (Fraser, 2008; Honneth, 1995). The indicatorization of justice can depoliticize it, turning radical demands into policy bite-sized objectives. Furthermore, the process of quantification is often more amenable to what is easily countable, and pushes aside more relational, complex, or emotional aspects of justice: dignity, recognition, or trauma. This "tyranny of indicators," as Muller (2018) puts it, can lead to moral reductionism, where the ethical richness of justice is narrowed into performance metrics. In fact, when governments declare "justice has been enhanced" due to the achievement of a statistical benchmark, they can close down collective criticism when injustice is still experienced in everyday life. This leads to a more fundamental question: are we in danger of taming justice, of draining it of its emancipatory power, by making it operational? Therefore, although indicators may serve justice they can also undermine its radical and ethical role; a threat which requires constant philosophical attention.

Hence, the turn to measure justice should be undertaken with methodological modesty and philosophical self-reflexivity. Justice indicators are not epistemic goals but bargained means, never not culturally, politically, and ethically context-free. They should not be crafted only to reflect the reality but to engage democratic conversation about what should be (Maurya, 2020). Justice, by its very nature, resists finalization. And any efforts to quantify it should seek to capture it in a manner that casts light on structural inequalities, gives voice to those marginalized, and avoid being seduced by the allure of simplistic numbers. Instead of necessarily giving up on justice as a social indicator because it is too complex, we need to celebrate that complexity, not as a symptom of failure, but as a symptom of moral seriousness.

Future Pathways and Recommendations

Justice needs to be seriously considered as a social indicator, not simply a rhetorical flourish in political speeches and manifestoes, and to achieve this it has to be theorized, operationalized, and integrated into the established framework of global and national indicators. By the above-mentioned philosophical inquiry, it is very much clear now that the normative validity and empirical feasibility of justice indicators, the future requires more than demonstration of concept. It needs a methodological revolution that is based on interdisciplinary cooperation, institutional integration, and ethical engagement.

Toward Institutional Integration: Justice in Global Frameworks

The first step toward legitimizing justice as a measurable indicator lies in embedding it into existing global frameworks such as the United Nations Development Programme (UNDP)'s Human Development Index (HDI), the Organisation for Economic Co-operation and Development (OECD)'s Better Life Index, and national well-being dashboards. Despite their conceptual richness, most current frameworks sideline justice. The HDI focuses on health, education, and income, but omits structural fairness or rights-based dimensions (UNDP, 2020). The OECD's How's Life? indicators include subjective well-being and civic engagement but lack a dedicated axis for justice (OECD, 2020). The omissions are not themselves incidental, they represent an unspoken belief that justice is either too amorphous to measure or too political to be made routine. But such assumptions are no longer tenable. As argued by Merry (2011), the global governance apparatus has already embraced indicators in sensitive areas like human rights and gender violence. Justice must be given similar attention, especially as a determinant of institutional legitimacy and predictor of social cohesion (Tyler, 2006). These global indexes should introduce justice as a distinct pillar or cross-cutting theme with the following sub-indicators:

- Access to legal aid (institutional justice)
- Equity in political representation (recognitional justice)
- Public perceptions of fairness (procedural justice)
- Rates of successful discrimination claims (distributive justice)

Governments and international bodies should consider justice not as an abstract ideal, but as a measurable component of development, akin to poverty, education, or environment.

Interdisciplinary Collaboration: Philosophers, Data Scientists, and Policy-Makers

Measuring justice is not a task that can be assigned to statisticians or policy designers only. It necessitates a radically interdisciplinary perspective uniting the normative expertise of philosophers, the technical abilities of data scientists, and the practical knowledge of policy-makers. Philosophers are essential to explain the conceptual differences among different kinds of justice, distributive, procedural, recognitional, restorative, and to establish the normative bar that metrics have to clear. Their input prevents justice indicators from becoming empty formalities, ensuring they reflect moral depth rather than bureaucratic convenience (Fraser, 2008; Sen, 2009). Data scientists are able to model resilient, multifaceted indicators that take into consideration cultural difference and time-based evolution. Advances in machine learning, sentiment analysis, and big data make it possible to mine qualitative narratives of injustice, such as court transcripts or complaint records, and convert them into usable metrics (Maurya, 2022). On their part, policy-makers ensure that justice measures are not only adopted, but institutionalized such that they are used to guide budgetary allocations, resource allocation, and legal reform. It is also important that they design accountability measures to protect against metric manipulation or symbolic compliance. The new epistemic infrastructure of justice indicators should take the form of this triangle: ethics, analytics, and governance.

Participatory Justice Metrics and the Democratic Imperative

A central critique of existing metrics is that they often exclude the very people they aim to represent (Espeland & Stevens, 2008). Justice, however, is not a quantity that can be dispensed to people; it must be accomplished with people. That requires developing participatory metrics, where communities have a role in shaping what justice is, what a violation is, and how to use indicators. Such models are already being tested through projects such as the Open Government Partnership and Participedia, which can provide blueprints to inclusive indicator design:

Future justice dashboards should therefore integrate:

- Citizen juries to deliberate on justice priorities
- Crowdsourced data on perceived injustices
- Narrative-based indicators drawn from lived experiences

Participation does not only enhance contextual sensitivity, but also leads to democratic legitimacy where measurement becomes a kind of empowerment instead of technocratic domination.

Areas for Future Research and Development

Although there has been increasing interest, the social indicator of justice is under-theorized and under implemented. Several research avenues deserve urgent attention:

- Justice Dashboards: Pilot programs that collect justice indicators at a city, state, and national level to promote real-time policy-making.
- Longitudinal Justice Studies: The study of the ways in which the variation of justice perception or outcomes influence the stability of the society or the economic growth or the trust of the people over a period of time.
- Intersectionality Metrics: Creating instruments that track interlocking injustices by race, gender, class, and ability.

Global South Justice Models: Constructing indicators around local philosophies, including Ubuntu, Dharma, or Buen Vivir, instead of introducing Western liberal models. International funding agencies, universities, and government think tanks need to be in the assisting end of these initiatives and make it clear that justice is not a matter of luxury, it is rather a fundamental need in democratic development. The treatment of justice as a social indicator is the acknowledgment that justice is not just a moral ideal, it is a policy-relevant, empirically identifiable, and normatively essential aspect of the quality of life. The ways ahead should be based on institutional ambition, interdisciplinary cooperation, and grassroots involvement to convert this vision into a reality. As Sen (2009) reminds us, justice is not about achieving perfection but reducing manifest injustice (Maurya, 2024). Indicators are, then, tools of humility, not to boast of what we have accomplished, but to light the way we have failed, and more importantly, the way we can accomplish more.

Concluding Summary

The case of introducing justice as a fundamental social indicator is not just an academic suggestion, but a political, ethical and epistemological necessity. In the course of this chapter, we have determined that not only can justice be theoretically constitutional to the quality of life (QoL) paradigm, but also that it is methodologically plausible as a measurable, multidimensional construct. The very act of excluding justice from global indices like the Human Development Index (HDI) or the OECD's Better Life Index is not a matter of oversight, but a form of epistemic negligence, one that perpetuates an illusion of progress while muting the lived experience of injustice. As Sen (2009) convincingly argues, the goal of social policy should not be to attain an ideal justice system, but to reduce identifiable injustices. According to this pragmatist inclination, justice becomes a practical field, an area of intervention. The justice measurement, then, is not utopian, it is radically realism. It tries to hold institutions answerable to their normative commitments and to monitor whether the benefits and the burdens allocation in the society is in accord with the democracy.

In fact, justice is arguably more than another social indicator, it is the moral fabric upon which all other indicators find their meaning. What is the merit of increased income when it is systematically excluded? What is the sense of access to education that replicates structural privilege? Without justice, indicators become hollow metrics, vulnerable to what Espeland and Stevens (2008) call "reactivity," the process by which people conform to metrics rather than metrics reflecting reality. The emancipatory possibility of metrics of justice is precisely their potential to both diagnostics of structural inequality and avoid the reductionism of the utilitarian flatland. Unlike indicators such as GDP, which conceal distributive disparities, or even subjective well-being, which can normalize suffering under systemic injustice, justice metrics demand disaggregation, transparency, and recognition of historical wrongs (Fraser, 2008). They take measurement systems out of the realm of technical performance and into the space of moral critique, of democratic engagement (Maurya, 2025).

Furthermore, justice can become a strategic reform lever when it is incorporated in national statistics, international indices, and policy dashboards. As shown in our global case studies, ranging from procedural justice in the Nordic welfare states to caste-based legal redress mechanisms in India, justice indicators have the capacity to shape public priorities, mobilize civil society, and inform equitable governance (Huq & Ginsburg, 2018; Tyler, 2006). Of course, this endeavor is not without peril. Measures of justice may be politicized, oversimplified, or distorted culturally as explained in the critique section. Nonetheless these risks do not discredit the case of measurement, they are the appeals to more adequate and reflexive and participatory designs. The measurement does not eliminate the richness of justice; it formalizes the requirement of fairness.

When relating this argument to the larger theme of the book, justice as a social indicator of quality of life (QoL), we need merely repeat what has been said previously, namely, that the end goal is not to settle on a singular definition of justice, but to make it a locus of ongoing debate and empirical responsibility. In the same way that the quality of life (QoL) movement has tried to take leave of economic measures to embrace the richer aspects of human well-being, it must now also develop to see justice as not a peripheral, but a primary measure of well-being. Justice, we have seen, is not an abstraction but a quantifiable, conflictual, and essential aspect of social existence. It would be not only to reform our statistics, but to add justice to our core social indicators. Amid the rising inequalities, democratic regression, and mistrust of public institutions, the demand to measure justice is nothing short of the demand to reappropriate our shared ability to identify and strive toward the good society.

References

Alkire, S., & Santos, M. E. (2010). *Acute multidimensional poverty: A new index for developing countries*. OPHI Working Paper No. 38. Oxford University.

Aristotle. (2009). *Nicomachean Ethics* (W. D. Ross, Trans.). Oxford University Press.

Braithwaite, J. (2001). *Restorative justice and responsive regulation*. Oxford University Press.

Chilisa, B. (2012). *Indigenous research methodologies*. SAGE Publications.

Christensen, T., & Laegreid, P. (2007). The whole-of-government approach to public sector reform. *Public Administration Review, 67*(6), 1059–1066.

Crenshaw, K. (1991). Mapping the margins: Intersectionality, identity politics, and violence against women of color. *Stanford Law Review, 43*(6), 1241–1299.

Deshpande, A. (2013). *Affirmative action in India*. Oxford University Press.

Diener, E., Suh, E. M., Lucas, R. E., & Smith, H. L. (1999). Subjective Well-being: Three decades of progress. *Psychological Bulletin, 125*(2), 276–302. https://doi.org/10.1037/0033-2909.125.2.276

Espeland, W. N., & Stevens, M. L. (2008). A sociology of quantification. *European Journal of Sociology, 49*(3), 401–436.

Fraser, N. (2008). *Scales of justice: Reimagining political space in a globalizing world*. Polity.

Gade, C. B. N. (2012). What is Ubuntu? Different interpretations among south Africans of African descent. *South African Journal of Philosophy, 31*(3), 484–503.

Gavrielides, T. (2007). *Restorative justice theory and practice: Addressing the discrepancy*. European Institute for Crime Prevention and Control.

Guru, G. (2000). Dalits from margin to margin. *India International Centre Quarterly, 27*(2), 143–152.

Helliwell, J. F., Layard, R., Sachs, J., & De Neve, J.-E. (Eds.). (2020). *World happiness report 2020*. Sustainable Development Solutions Network.

Honneth, A. (1995). *The struggle for recognition: The moral grammar of social conflicts*. Polity Press.

HSRC (Human Sciences Research Council). (2020). *South African Social Attitudes Survey 2019*.

Huq, A. Z., & Ginsburg, T. (2018). How to lose constitutional democracy. *UCLA Law Review, 65*, 78–169.

IEP (Institute for Economics and Peace). (2023). *Global Peace Index 2023*. https://www.visionofhumanity.org
Land, K. C. (2001). Social indicators. In N. J. Smelser & P. B. Baltes (Eds.), *International encyclopedia of the social & behavioral sciences* (pp. 14706–14709). Elsevier.
Levi, M., Sacks, A., & Tyler, T. (2009). Conceptualizing legitimacy, measuring legitimating beliefs. *American Behavioral Scientist, 53*(3), 354–375.
Mamdani, M. (2002). Amnesty or impunity? A preliminary critique of the report of the truth and reconciliation Commission of South Africa (TRC). *Diacritics, 32*(3–4), 33–59.
Marmot, M. (2005). Social determinants of health inequalities. *The Lancet, 365*(9464), 1099–1104. https://doi.org/10.1016/S0140-6736(05)71146-6
Maurya, S. K. (2020). A reply to Louis P. Pojman's article "the case against affirmative action.". *Conatus—Journal of Philosophy, 5*(2), 87–113.
Maurya, S. K. (2021). The concept of justice in reference with philosophies of Plato and Aristotle: A critical study. *Journal of Liberty and International Affairs, 7*(3), 250–266. https://doi.org/10.47305/JLIA21370250m
Maurya, S. K. (2022). On just, justice and distributive justice: A critical and comparative discourse. *Journal of Liberty and International Affairs, 8*(2), 240–254. https://doi.org/10.47305/JLIA2282240m
Maurya, S. K. (2024). African philosophies of justice and equity: A contemporary discourse. *African Journal of Religion, Philosophy and Culture, 5*(2), 61–78. https://doi.org/10.31920/2634-7644/2024/v5n2a4
Maurya, S. K. (2025). Restorative justice and karmic justice: Ubuntu and Vedanta in dialogue. *African Journal of Religion, Philosophy and Culture, 6*(2).
Merry, S. E. (2011). Measuring the world: Indicators, human rights, and global governance. *Current Anthropology, 52*(S3), S83–S95.
Merry, S. E. (2016). *The seductions of quantification: Measuring human rights, gender violence, and sex trafficking*. University of Chicago Press.
Muller, J. Z. (2018). *The tyranny of metrics*. Princeton University Press.
Noll, H. H. (2002). Towards a European system of social indicators: Theoretical framework and system architecture. *Social Indicators Research, 58*(1–3), 47–87.
Nussbaum, M. C. (2011). *Creating capabilities: The human development approach*. Harvard University Press.
OECD. (2019). *Government at a glance*. OECD Publishing.
OECD. (2020). *How's life? 2020: Measuring Well-being*. OECD Publishing.
OECD. (2021). *Access to justice and legal empowerment: A synthesis report*. OECD Publishing.
OHCHR. (2012). *Human rights indicators: A guide to measurement and implementation*. United Nations.
Pande, R. (2003). Can mandated political representation increase policy influence for disadvantaged minorities? Theory and evidence from India. *American Economic Review, 93*(4), 1132–1151.
Pew Research Center. (2020). *Public trust in government: 1958–2020*. https://www.pewresearch.org
Rawls, J. (1971). *A theory of justice*. Harvard University Press.
Rawls, J. (1993). *Political liberalism*. Columbia University Press.
Republic of South Africa. (1996). *The Constitution of the Republic of South Africa*.
Rothstein, B. (2005). *Social traps and the problem of trust*. Cambridge University Press.
Sen, A. (1993). Capability and Well-being. In M. C. Nussbaum & A. Sen (Eds.), *The quality of life* (pp. 30–53). Oxford University Press.
Sen, A. (2009). *The idea of justice*. Harvard University Press.
Smith, L. T. (1999). *Decolonizing methodologies: Research and indigenous peoples*. Zed Books.
Sowell, T. (2004). *Affirmative action around the world: An empirical study*. Yale University Press.
Thorat, S., & Newman, K. S. (2012). *Blocked by caste: Economic discrimination in modern India*. Oxford University Press.

Transparency International. (2022). *Corruption Perceptions Index 2022.*
Tyler, T. R. (2006). *Why people obey the law* (2nd ed.). Princeton University Press.
UNDP. (1990). *Human Development Report 1990*. Oxford University Press.
UNDP. (2009). *Programming for justice: Access for all*. United Nations Development Programme.
UNDP. (2020). *Human development report 2020: The next frontier*. United Nations Development Programme.
World Bank. (2022). South Africa economic update.
World Justice Project. (2023). *Rule of Law Index 2023*. https://worldjusticeproject.org
Young, I. M. (1990). *Justice and the politics of difference*. Princeton University Press.

Chapter 5
Empirical Studies Linking Justice and Well-Being

Introduction: The Normative-Empirical Nexus

Justice has been one of the cornerstones of philosophical discourse, it functions as a vital ideal along which the society is judged, and in which claims which are moral are authenticated. From Plato's tripartite conception of harmony in the soul and polis to Rawls's formulation of "justice as fairness" (Rawls, 1971), philosophical theories have approached justice as a normative benchmark, abstract, evaluative, and often aspirational. However, the late twentieth and early twenty-first centuries have seen a decisive turn toward empirical approaches to the study of justice, which attempt to bridge the gap between justice and life experience, quantifiable well-being, and policy outcome. The shift poses deep philosophical concerns regarding the connection between the normative ideals and the empirical realities. As Amartya Sen has emphasized, justice must not remain imprisoned in ideal theory but must confront "the injustices that people have reason to resent" in their actual lives (Sen, 2009, p. vii). It is not merely a positivist impulse that demands that justice should be expressible in observable signs, and the moral pressure here is that justice should illumine the lights and shadows of the empirical world so that it can be judged and argued about. But this is the main paradox of the chapter and of the book in truth: how is a value so normatively thick, so context-sensitive, so interpretively rich as justice to be the object of empirical inquiry without becoming distorted or reduced? This is an issue that has demanded continued interest beyond the design and interpretation of social indicators beyond the epistemological underpinnings on which traditions of empiricism are grounded.

S. K. Maurya, *Exploring Justice as a Social Indicator of Life*, Social Indicators Research Series 92, https://doi.org/10.1007/978-3-032-10812-8_5

From Philosophical Ideal to Lived Condition

Traditionally understood as relating to rights, fairness, equality, and recognition, justice is not just a regulative notion, but simultaneously it is a form of embodied relationship. People and societies are not exposed to justice and injustice, abstractly but in the dealings they grapple with materially, in their symbolic recognition, and their interaction with institutes. This necessitates that justice should be empirically debated to be morally sensitive and politically effective. Empirical research can, for instance, uncover how perceptions of distributive and procedural justice affect trust in institutions, willingness to cooperate, and subjective well-being (Tyler, 2006; Helliwell & Putnam, 2004). It can reveal structural patterns of injustice that elude philosophical abstraction, such as the intersection of race, class, and geography in health care access, or the gendered dimensions of unpaid care work (Folbre, 2001). This information is always, of course, morally noncomprehensive, but it enriches the philosophical investigations on the basis of the moral phenomenology of realized life. This empirical engagement should however be done with philosophical vigilance. Yet, not everything that can be measured is important, and not everything that is important can be easily measured. The threat of instrumentalism of justice, that is, turning it into strands of technocratic measures, should be countered with the promise of epistemic self-reflexivity and normative coherence.

Well-Being as an Ethically Loaded Construct

It is an empirical working on the justice that is frequently sought out by its alleged influences on well-being? Whenever it is defined in terms of happiness, life satisfaction, capabilities, or functioning well-being invites a set of philosophical suppositions about what the good life is. Moreover, utilitarian conceptions such as well-being can be reduced to pleasure or utility, which lure aggregation and maximization. But as critics such as Martha Nussbaum (2012) and Elizabeth Anderson (1995) argue, such views neglect the qualitative plurality of human values and the moral significance of agency, dignity, and recognition. Subjective well-being measures, while appealing for their simplicity, are vulnerable to adaptive preferences, where individuals internalize unjust conditions and report satisfaction within constrained choices (Sen, 1985). Even more sophisticated metrics such as the Human Development Index (HDI) or the Multidimensional Poverty Index (MPI) rest on normative decisions about which dimensions to include, how to weigh them, and whose perspectives count. These are not empirically based decisions but morally built—these are based on judgment concerning human flourishing, moral significance, and social priority. This means that the empirical equivalents of justice have to be placed under the never-ending philosophical examination. They must not only reflect existing preferences but also open space for critical evaluation of those preferences—especially when they emerge from contexts of deprivation, marginalization, or epistemic injustice (Fricker, 2007).

The Potential and Dangers of Combining Normative Justice and Empirical Evidence

The combination of justice and empirical data has great potential: it can set out to diagnose latent injustices, judge the effects of policy, and activate discourse. Social indicators, when employed ethically, can be used to improve transparency, democratic accountability, and institutional responsiveness. They are able to become a tool of criticism that reveals the disjuncture between ideals and institutions. However, this integration is fraught with philosophical peril. First, it risks what Nancy Cartwright (2007) calls the "thinness of models": the oversimplification of complex moral realities into indicators that obscure more than they reveal. Second, it invites what Michael Power (1997) terms the "audit culture," where the demand for measurement replaces substantive ethical engagement with procedural compliance. Third, it can unwittingly reproduce epistemic domination, privileging elite knowledge systems and excluding vernacular or subaltern understandings of justice (Santos, 2014). To enable itself to navigate through these risks, a philosophy of measurement needs to be put into words, and this philosophy needs to be one that accepts epistemic pluralism, methodological humility, and normative transparency. Indications ought not to be considered as absolute facts but as temporary replenishments, as is always subject to challenge, change, reinterpretation.

The empirical study of justice and well-being has engaged several disciplinary traditions that exhibit different methodological instruments and epistemic premises. The welfare economics and economics as a whole has tried to measure and quantify well-being by utility, income, or consumption. The emergence of behavioral economics and happiness studies has complicated this picture, introducing psychological insights into preferences, adaptation, and heuristics (Kahneman & Deaton, 2010). Nonetheless, those methods can be context-free and are often impersonal and discriminating of individuals as subjects of preferences, as opposed to normatively located agents. There have been contributions of measures on subjective well-being, life satisfaction, and resilience by psychology, particularly positive psychology. Although laden with phenomenological wisdom, these steps may personalize structural as well as ethical issues and transfer the injustice to the way of thinking instead of concentrating on institutional faults. Sociology puts a spotlight on social systems, norms, and institutions providing means of examining recognition, status, and inequality based on groups. The attention that it draws toward relational and symbolic aspects of injustice supplements distributive accounts, even though much of the analysis is nonnormative. Development studies and public policy are processes that run along the boundaries of empirical and ethical assessments. Following the popularization of Capability Approach proposed by Sen, more and more of this kind of field uses multidimensional indexes to measure complex deprivation and empowerment. It is, perhaps, here that philosophical dialogue has been most fruitful with empiricism. Even in this case, there are some methodological issues to be solved: to compare the capabilities across different contexts, to aggregate in the face of value pluralism, and to provide participatory validity. They are not just technical questions, but strong philosophical questions, requiring us to be clear about what we are valuing, why we are valuing it, and how we should behave on that valuation.

Justice and Subjective Well-Being: Correlational and Causal Claims

The empirical study of well-being has experienced a paradigmatic shift in its investigation in recent decades. No longer confined to income, consumption, or utility, contemporary frameworks increasingly embrace subjective well-being (SWB)-an individual's self-assessed life satisfaction and emotional experiences, as a major proxy for the quality of life. At the same time, the notion of justice has shifted toward being more institutional toward perceptions, feelings, and expectations of justice, rights, and recognition. The intersection begs a critical question: what degree to which individual sense of justice has an impact on subject well-being and what such a correlation tells us about the moral aspects of human flourishing. This question is more than a simple instance of correlation. This empirical correlation between justice and well-being has implications on the philosophical arguments over whether justice is in fact a good, and, to what extent an institution creates a context where we flourish as human beings, and whether the hedonic metrics used actually have sufficient normative depth to the human experience. This chapter critically examines the significant results of cross-national polls, actual experiments, and psychological theories with placing the results in the context of philosophically consistent interpretation of the subjective well-being as constructs of ethical type. Large-scale international surveys such as the World Values Survey (WVS) and the Gallup World Poll have provided compelling, though uneven, evidence for the proposition that perceptions of justice are significantly correlated with subjective well-being. The Gallup data, for example, show that individuals who report confidence in judicial systems and trust in fairness of public institutions consistently report higher levels of life satisfaction, even when controlling for income, education, and employment status (Gallup, 2023). Similarly, WVS respondents who affirm that their societies are "run in the interests of all" rather than "for a few powerful groups" tend to score higher on happiness indices.

These discoveries give credence to the fact that subjective justice or how people perceive that they are treated fairly is very significant to their perception regarding their lives. This empirical link challenges older liberal theories which, following Rawls, emphasized the "priority of the right over the good" (Rawls, 1971, p. 31), suggesting instead that fairness is internal to the very conception of well-being. Nevertheless, there are also cultural and ideological mediations of the justice, well-being relationship provided by such surveys. In some authoritarian or collectivist societies, respondents report high satisfaction despite systemic injustices, possibly due to adaptive preferences or norm internalization (Sen, 1985). This brings in the possibility of subjective satisfactions being an unreliable substitute to objective justice and whether it is normatively acceptable to have high SWB among those who live in unjust societies. In addition to these general associations, there is an expanding empirical literature that investigated how perceptions of justice impact well-being through their mechanisms of action. One of the critical mediating variables in this relationship is institutional trust. In their landmark studies, Helliwell and Putnam (2004) argue that trust in legal and political institutions is not merely a reflection of well-being but a substantive contributor to it. Their regression analyses indicate that trust, and especially trust based on procedural fairness perceptions, is a better indicator of happiness than income even health.

(Helliwell et al., 2018). These are relational and psychological goods whose direct contribution is subjective life evaluations. Nevertheless, normative asymmetry does exist: institutional trust can increase subjective well-being, but it is not associated with justice. People can be satisfied with the belief in the systems of great injustice. The given phenomenon demonstrates the need to subject the empirical results to the philosophical scrutiny: the subjective trust has to be balanced not only with the returns of hedonic satisfaction but also with the ethical appropriateness of the trusted object in itself.

Experimental and Longitudinal Studies on Procedural Justice

The causal argument gets reinforced with the procedural justice tradition pioneered by Tom R. Tyler in the field of experimental psychology. The experiments and longitudinal research carried by Tyler provide evidence that procedural fairness ascertains outcome acceptance regardless of material outcomes- individuals abide by unfavourable decisions when they believe the procedure was fair, either in a legal, workplace, or bureaucratic context (Tyler & Blader, 2003). This understanding has far-reaching consequences in terms of how to go about the designing of public institutions. Insofar as it places procedural justice beyond just instrumental effectiveness to containing within it a sense of intuitively good-in-itself, it harmonizes with Rawlsian and Habermasian commitments to the reasons of the public and respectful reciprocity. Participants in Tyler's studies consistently report greater well-being, institutional satisfaction, and civic engagement when they feel they were heard, respected, and treated with neutrality. These findings also intersect with recent work in social neuroscience showing that fair treatment activates reward-related brain regions, whereas perceptions of injustice correlate with heightened stress and reduced affective well-being. This is strengthened by the psychophysiological evidence that states that justice is not a supra-embodied norm but a subjective experience, somatically and emotionally. Though, the very psychological orientation to subjective perceptions is an invitation to philosophic questioning. Is perceived fairness equivalent to real fairness? Is it possible to say that procedural justice is morally sufficient without the proper outcomes? And will the desire to acquiesce in less-than-just results in the interest of procedural rectitude have the effect of providing justification to structural injustice?

Hedonic Versus Eudaimonic Well-Being: Philosophical Challenges

One of the major criticisms of subjective well-being as a measure of justice flows out of the division between hedonic and eudaimonic conceptions of the good life. Hedonic approaches, dominant in much of the SWB literature, equate well-being with pleasure maximization and pain minimization, measured via affective balance and life satisfaction scales (Diener et al., 1999). In contrast, eudaimonic approaches, rooted in Aristotelian virtue ethics, define well-being as living in accordance with one's values, fulfilling human potential, and exercising agency in a just society (Nussbaum, 2012; Ryff & Singer, 1998). On this account, subjective happiness is in no wise needed or sufficient to well-being. It is possible to be content with a situation that is highly unjust because of the factors of adaptation, misrecognition, or internalized oppression. On the other hand, the sufferer can be affected when seeking justice in unjust circumstances, an experience that is common to those who are activists, whistleblowers, and critics of the society. As Nussbaum (2013) observes, "being angry at injustice, grieving for others' pain, or being outraged by cruelty" are not signs of ill-being but expressions of moral integrity (p. 31). Moreover, cross-cultural research reveals that subjective well-being norms are themselves culturally specific, shaped by narratives of individualism, stoicism, or social harmony (Christopher, 1999). Therefore, the use of SWB as a uniform index of justice comes at the risk of both ethical ethnocentrism and epistemic injustice. The evidence indicates that justice is a significant variable in how individuals perceive, reason and how they treat one another. However, there is the expression of the warning that an oversimplified equation of subjective well-being could be reduced to social conditions solely. It requires critical reflective empiricism: the tendency to respect an experienced situation and not to confuse the inclination to comfort with the inclination to justice or contentedness with the inclination to legitimacy. This method should question the moral valence of subjective means: do they result in fair observation or they are products of unfair compromise? It should evaluate the institutional realities that precondition perceptions: are they actually just or just appear just? It needs to be open to eudaimonic measures, like capabilities, dignity, and moral agency, which more effectively embrace the moral complexity of human flourishing. In philosophical terms, empirical research on justice and well-being does not reduce justice and data. They give justice, rather, in the lived experience, in materializing moral assertions by projecting them into the tragedy, struggle and hopes of real individuals.

Distributive Justice and Economic Inequality

The central question of the theory of justice of the classical theory as well as in modern theory of justice is that of distribution, the question of how goods, opportunities, and burdens have to be distributed over individuals and groups within a society. Distributive justice has always been a normative issue: whether the Aristotelian principle of proportionality or the Rawlsian difference principle, the issue has always been whether the distribution of goods corresponds to normative theories of distributive justice. The last few decades, though, have seen a new wave of empirical studies, which purport to associate distributive outcomes and especially income inequality with tangible measures of societal well-being. The notable work is *The Spirit Level: Why More Equal Societies Almost Always Do Better* by Richard Wilkinson and Kate Pickett (2009) that brought up debate across the globe by stating that less unequal societies always perform better in health, prevention of crimes, education, and social trust.

However, though there is empirical salience to such claims, the philosophical ramifications thereof are debatable. Are egalitarian societies simply better at producing utilitarian results, or are they more just societies? Is it possible to separate empirically measured evils of inequality with cultural, institutional, and ideological mediations? This chapter examines the philosophical stakes of empirical research in the field of economic inequality, both in terms of what such research concludes, and in terms of what it presupposes normatively (Michalos & Hatch, 2020).

Empirical Links Between Inequality and Social Pathologies

Income inequality is often linked to a range of social issues, including poor physical and mental health, higher crime rates, drug abuse, lower educational attainment, limited social mobility, and decreased levels of interpersonal trust. With regard to the bottom half, they argue its main point simply, namely, that unequal societies, all things considered, nearly always fare rather poorly on a broad variety of indicators of quality of life, not just among the poor, but at all levels of income. This argument is supported by substantial empirical evidence. The same sample findings, based on OECD, World Bank, and WHO data, show that the poorer quality of results, an outcome lower life expectancy, increased incarceration, an overly polarized politics, etc uphold the high-inequality nations (those with higher Gini coefficients) such as USA and UK over and above their more egalitarian strong foes such as Sweden, Norway, and Japan.(OECD, 2021a, 2021b). It is psychosocial and structural:

inequality causes or contributes to chronic stress, social erosion, and erosion of the public goods of flourishing. Furthermore, income inequality has been empirically linked to erosions in institutional trust and civic participation, which in turn have downstream effects on subjective well-being and democratic legitimacy (Putnam, 2000; Helliwell & Huang, 2008). These findings resonate with Rawlsian intuitions about the role of justice in maintaining the "basic structure" of society and its effect on citizens' self-respect and moral development (Rawls, 1971, §79).

Critiques: Causal Ambiguity and Cultural Mediation

In spite of the scope of empirical correlations, methodological and philosophical objections criticize the explanation of such results. First is the issue of causality. The relationship between inequality and bad outcomes is not causative. According to the skeptics, there is a chance that third variables, including but not limited to cultural attitudes toward authority, historical trends of segregation, or religious adherence rates, mediated or confounded the relationship between inequality and the malfunction of social life (Lynch et al., 2004). Moreover, countries with high inequality but extensive welfare protections (e.g., France) do not always follow the predicted pattern, suggesting that policy mediates the impact of inequality. Analogously, understood injustices in society may be a matter of deep-rooted structural injustice even in the societies whose level of measured inequality is relatively low, a fact testified by the existence of castes, exclusion of races, or discrimination in the law, which should question the sufficiency of the income-based measures on their own. Second is the issue of cultural mediation. Empirical researches tend to presume that all the evils of inequality are universalistic and the same in terms of psychology. But anthropological studies reveal that the normative relevance of inequality is different in different cultures. In certain East Asian cultures, such as East Asia, hierarchical differences have been less pathologized because of the Confucianism beliefs that equate hierarchical order as orderly and virtuous. Elsewhere, inequality can be excused where it is carried out as meritocratic or morally deserved and this emphasizes the significance of perceptions of justice compared to details of income inequality. All these criticisms indicate a more serious problem: that which is to be taken as injustice cannot be read out of empirical data solely. That inequality has negative consequences does not make it unjust; and its negative consequences would not justify inequality escaping its moral costs. As Sen (2009) emphasizes, justice is not reducible to outcomes, it is also about processes, opportunities, and respect for persons.

Cross-National Comparisons: Nordic Versus Anglo-American Models

The sharpest clarifications of the empirical comparison are probably the one between the Nordic social democracies and Anglo-American liberal market economies. The former exhibit lower levels of income inequality, higher trust in government, more generous social protections, and higher average scores on both subjective well-being and equality of opportunity (Esping-Andersen, 1990; OECD, 2021a, 2021b). Conversely, nations such as the USA and UK boast of sharp wealth gradients, stratified public services, and deteriorating intergenerational mobility. These empirical differences have been taken two contradicting ways. Egalitarian thesis assumes that just institutions lead to just outcomes, and that common achievement of Nordic nations indicates a more profound sense of endorsement to open-mindedness, solidarity, and human decency. According to this opinion, they do not just work efficiently but demonstrate a model of how things should be done morally as Rawls or Sen would have imagined justice that is both about fairness and the nurture of capacity. Alternatively, the policy artifact thesis is that differences are historically contingent, and institutionally constructed, and not manifestations of moral superiority. Based on this interpretation, Nordic performance is a cause of good bureaucracies, political homogeneity, and past histories characterized by low corruption rather than stronger justice engulfs. In that case, their effective performance might be hard to imitate in more pluralistic, diverse, or federal structures.

The philosophic question, next, is whether we may conclude to normative legitimacy on account of empirical efficacy. Due to the greater performance of the egalitarian societies, is it more just to be an egalitarian society or the society that is more just is the one that is performing better due to a contingent circumstance? This distinction is not semantic. It also poses a pertinent question on the parameters according to which justice is to be considered, instrumental utility, procedural justice, or substantive equality.

Philosophical Stakes: Efficiency or Justice?

The thought that distributive justice and empirical social science need to converge sets a more underlying philosophical conundrum: are egalitarian policies justified by the fact that they lead to well-being or does justification lie in internal moral commitments to fairness, dignity, and non-domination? Equality, according to utilitarianism, could only be endorsed by the generation of aggregate well-being. Redistribution is considered acceptable on such a view as a way to a hedonic end. Such a rationale can be seen as morally inadequate, though, as seen in a Kantian or Rawlsian light. Injustice does not involve the maximization of good outcomes: It is a failure to treat persons as ends in themselves and on reasonable terms of cooperation, with free and equal citizens. Indeed, if inequality were someday shown to increase aggregate happiness (e.g., by incentivizing innovation or growth), would we still endorse it? The liberal-egalitarian response would be that the answer is no: justice is not servant to consequence. Equality is not merely desirable as it contributes to more favorable results, but rather it reflects on the moral value of people that are equal.

Meanwhile, the fact that justice claims have to be empirically verified is not immaterial. Provided that inequality is proved to deteriorate health, divide communities, and make social mobility even more unlikely, this is not the simple statement of the facts of the matter, but the moral condemnation of the systems that do not accomplish the prerequisites of the human flourishing. As Elizabeth Anderson (1999) argues, equality must be understood not only in terms of resource distribution but in terms of relational and democratic ideals: who counts, who decides, who is heard. The empirical science bill of the literature on inequality, health, and well-being has come out strongly in advancement of the argument that says inequality is harmful to societies on ethical, psychological, and institutional levels. However, these results cannot be treated in a morally autonomous way. An instrumental effectiveness of egalitarian justice may not be the only support of philosophical argument of egalitarian justice. Justice should also have its normative commitment premises in concepts of freedom, dignity, recognition, and solidarity. It is one thing to have a more integrated appreciation of distributive justice and another to give up on empirical insights and also the attempt to reduce ethics to economics. Instead, we need to make room for philosophically adept empiricism: empiricism that will reveal hitherto un-detected harms, verify moral intuitions, and inform institutional reform, without being hostage to considerations of statistical significance.

Recognition, Social Identity, and Psychological Well-Being

Though there exist a body of empirical work addressing issues of justice, much of which has involved work on distributive types of inequalities, navigating this empirical landscape also seems to have become a domain on the justice foundational grounds, bound by one very crucial and under-theorized aspect of justice that concerning recognition. The recognition paradigm, articulated most robustly by Axel Honneth (1995), posits that human flourishing depends not only on the equitable distribution of resources, but also on the affirmation of identity, dignity, and social worth. The stigmatization, the rejection, the humiliation, in short, the symbolic violence that is misrecognition, is not an insult in the moral sense but a deformation of the self and a debasing of the well-being. These arguments are empirically proving to be more accurate indeed, recent interdisciplinary studies, especially those in social psychology, public health, and critical theory are finding that recognition deficit results in psychological damage, identity death, and decline in mental health. The current section addresses the intersection of recognition theory and empirical research on social identity, marginalization, and well-being. It claims that recognition is not incidentally a soft moral consideration but a constitutive constituent of psychological integrity and the salient measure in the test of fairness of the social institutions.

Recognition, Misrecognition, and the Self: Honneth's Normative Framework

Axel Honneth's *The Struggle for Recognition* (1995) extends Hegelian and Habermasian traditions to formulate a normative theory of justice grounded in intersubjective recognition. On the one hand, Honneth asserts the self to be a socially constituted identity, conceived together with its relations of love, rights, and solidarity, and not an isolated monad as in Kant. These three spheres of recognition correspond, respectively, to primary relationships (affection), legal standing (respect), and social esteem (value contribution). In this schema, recognition is the precondition of autonomy. Without this recognition, people can only experience what Honneth defines as identity damage, a kind of moral and psychological injury, which affects the ability to connect with others and themselves as a free and equal agent. Misrecognition therefore amounts to both an ethical and a pathogenic condition, structurally implanted in the mechanisms of injustice. Notably, the Honneth theory tends to oppose the clash of material versus symbolic harms. Justice is not just a matter of distribution supplemented by recognition, recognition is an organizational aspect of justice that establishes whose lives matter, whose voices will be heard, and whose cries will be recognized. Empirical research on stigma, social exclusion, and psychological suffering has echoed these findings particularly among the marginalized.

Empirical Evidence of Recognition Theory: Stigma, Exclusion, and Identity Harm

The psychological costs of misrecognition explained by Honneth have been confirmed in more recent years by social psychological studies. Studies on stigma, particularly the work of Erving Goffman (1963) and its subsequent developments in the health sciences, demonstrate that individuals subjected to devalued identities experience chronic stress, diminished self-esteem, and internalized shame. For example, Link and Phelan (2001) identify stigma as a process that links labeling, stereotyping, and status loss, culminating in discriminatory outcomes that harm psychological well-being. Further empirical evidence comes from research on social exclusion, which has been shown to activate brain regions associated with physical pain (Eisenberger et al., 2003). This reinforces the point that being ignored, dismissed, or excluded is neurobiologically real, as opposed to metaphorical, which is what Honneth most likely would suggest when he argues that recognition is constitutive of human dignity.

Additionally, identity-based exclusion, such as homophobia, Islamophobia, or ableism, has been correlated with higher rates of anxiety, depression, and suicidality (Meyer, 2003). These consequences are more than mental health statistics; they are moral facts, showing the psychic price of a society which denies difference recognition.

Marginalization and Mental Health: Race, Gender, and Caste

The consequences of the lack of recognition are especially sharp when it comes to structural marginalization around the denial of symbolic legitimacy to whole groups of people. Critical race theory, feminist psychology, and Dalit studies have developed empirical lineages broadly proving the connection between racial, gendered, and caste-based misrecognition and psychological distress. In the USA, for example, Black Americans face disproportionately high rates of hypertension, PTSD, and clinical depression, attributable not solely to material deprivation but to the everyday burdens of racial stigma, stereotype threat, and cultural devaluation. These findings lend empirical support to Frantz Fanon's (1952) theorization of colonial alienation and internalized inferiority, which he famously described as "epidermalized inferiority." Similarly, feminist scholars have documented how gender-based misrecognition, including sexual objectification, workplace discrimination, and erasure in public discourse, contributes to body image disorders, chronic anxiety, and reduced life satisfaction (Bartky, 1990; Fredrickson & Roberts, 1997). In South Asia, Dalit also experience caste-based ostracization, which is realized not only in the access to resources but also the human being itself. It has been empirically demonstrated that humiliation in schools, temples, and healthcare environments causes an increase in dropout rates, poor health outcomes, and intergenerational trauma. These trends show that symbolic degradation is frequently the reflection of material inequality, and that justice needs to correct it.

Psychological Correlates of Just Treatment: Dignity, Respect, and Agency

The recognition theory also highlights the positive aspects of justice: what occurs when people are affirmed, treated respectfully, and related as equals. In this case, psychological well-being and agency are particularly relevant as the subject of empirical studies. Carol Ryff's multidimensional model of well-being, for instance, identifies autonomy, positive relations, and purpose in life as core components, dimensions that resonate strongly with Honneth's model of recognitional autonomy (Ryff & Singer, 1998). Research has shown that individuals who report being treated with dignity and respect by public institutions, such as police, courts, and social services, are more likely to exhibit resilience, civic trust, and a sense of belonging (Tyler, 2006). These results support literature on procedural justice and would allow a nonutilitarian argument in favor of democratic involvement: the fact of being heard, even in the absence of adoption of preferences, is a source of psychological recognition and political empowerment. These findings defy the logic that well-being is a product of outcomes in itself. Instead, they argue that fair treatment equals respect and moral consideration, which is reciprocated and leads to psychosocial values that cannot be replaced by material goods.

Moral Injury, Collective Trauma, and Post-Conflict Injustice

One last area of empirical investigation that has proven particularly fruitful with regard to the theory of recognition is the investigation of moral injury and collective trauma. Originating in military psychology, the concept of moral injury refers to the psychological distress that results from betrayal or participation in morally transgressive acts (Litz et al., 2009). The victims of torture, genocide, or state violence are usually tormented not only by PTSD but by the destruction of moral ego and social identity. Qualitative research in post-conflict societies, such as Rwanda, Bosnia, and South Africa, shows that truth-telling, public acknowledgment, and reparative rituals are essential not only for political reconciliation but for restoring individual and communal identities. Such practices are not merely cathartic, they are forms of re-recognition, through which victims are affirmed as moral beings whose pain is important. Appreciation is needed in these situations and this need can be more pressing than financial rewards. As Judith Butler (2004) argues, "recognition is not a reward we grant the human, but the condition under which the human becomes possible" (p. 2). In this sense, justice is the process by which subjectivity is reconstructed after social annihilation.

What was once deemed too soft to investigate in an empirical way has become a critical perspective through which we analyze the psychological and moral aspects of justice. And both empirical research in all fields of inquiry and theoretical arguments are growing in support of the claims that being an identity, enjoying dignity, and possessing social esteem are not only subjective preferences, but also normatively charged and psychologically required goods. A theory of justice based on recognition criticizes utilitarian explanations of justice that place primary emphasis on aggregate welfare and liberal theories that marginalize the cultural and symbolic aspects of harm. It requires that measures of well-being must not only focus onincome or happiness, but also on respect, inclusion, and affirmation. What matters more is that it requires institutional changes that no longer regard recognition as an act of toleration but rather structural necessity, on which and through which people can live, act, and thrive as moral equals.

Institutional Trust, Justice, and Democratic Participation

Whether the populace actually trusts the outcome of a democratic institution is not the only principle that determines its legitimacy, it is also the perceived fairness of the process and participation that determines the legitimacy of democratic institutions. This observation, once casually dismissed by political philosophers according to Rawls or Habermas, is increasingly being bolstered by the literature on procedural justice, which holds that it is not the quality of decisions per se that determines how people comply with them, how people trust and engage with them but how such decisions are arrived at. Procedural justice, in this context, is not reducible to mere rule-following; it concerns the normative and affective dimensions of institutional authority, including voice, neutrality, transparency, and dignity (Tyler, 2006)

Procedural Justice and Civic Trust: Empirical Evidence

The connection between perceived procedural fairness and trust in the public institution has also been observationally confirmed in social psychology and political science. Tom R. Tyler's pioneering research (1990; 2006) shows that individuals are more likely to accept and comply with legal decisions, even unfavorable ones, if they believe the process was fair, impartial, and respectful. The ideal of procedural justice, according to this perspective, is not an extravagance but a civic virtue: it creates the perception that one is both a valued actor in a common moral project, rather than a subject of a bureaucratic edict. The results achieved by Tyler have been duplicated and further developed by subsequent researchers in various settings: court systems, policing, tax compliance, delivery of public services, and organizational governance.

At the macro-level, survey data from the World Justice Project and OECD's Trust in Government initiative confirm that perceived fairness, transparency, and impartiality in governance are strong predictors of public trust, civic engagement, and social cohesion (OECD, 2021a, 2021b; World Justice Project, 2023). The citizens in societies whose justice systems are perceived to be corrupt or biased have less institutional legitimacy, despite better outcomes. The findings discredit instrumentalist theories of governance that hold efficiency or performance as central to governance rather than process. Instead, they indicate that procedural justice offers its own, unique source of legitimacy, which is based on mutual recognition and moral reciprocity.

Legal Empowerment and Access to Justice

The global community and institutions, such as the UNDP and the World Bank, have promoted the concept of legal empowerment to incorporate the agency of marginalized groups to interpret, enjoy, and creatively engage the law in procedural justice. Legal empowerment reframes access to justice not as access to courts per se, but as the ability to claim rights, resolve disputes, and influence decision-making through participatory mechanisms (UNDP, 2016). Empirical studies in India, Kenya, and the Philippines, for instance, have shown that community paralegal programs, legal literacy campaigns, and participatory land adjudication increase not only legal awareness but also civic trust and political efficacy. The respondents indicate increased readiness to deal with the state, decreased fear of law agencies, and enhanced unity in solving societal problems. The normative import of these findings lies in their affirmation of Amartya Sen's capabilities approach to justice: legal procedures are not merely instruments for conflict resolution; they are means of expanding individual and collective agency (Sen, 2009). In this sense justice is achieved not just in verdicts but also in procedures that renew voice, dignity, and deliberative inclusion.

Democratic Legitimacy and Fairness in Allocation: Experimental Insights

On the academic terrain of democratic theory, the experimental economics has provided high-valued information on how preconceptions of justice determine tendency to cooperation, trust, and legitimacy. The public goods games, ultimatum games and dictator games have always demonstrated that people are more apt to contribute to collective welfare where they trust allocation mechanisms to be fair and so even at personal expense (Fehr & Gächter, 2000). For example, participants are more likely to accept unequal distributions when the procedure for determining them is transparent and inclusive. On the contrary, untransparent or capricious procedures provoke feelings of resentment, nonadherence, and vindictive actions irrespective of the material rewards granted. These findings mirror John Rawls's (1971) argument that fair processes are essential to the legitimacy of distributive outcomes, even when inequalities are permitted under the difference principle. Furthermore, due to the principles of deliberative legitimacy, which is one of the tenets of Habermasian discourse ethics, there is fairness in decision-making. The willingness to abide by a collective decision hinges not on its substance alone, but on whether it emerged through procedures that respect each participant as a rational and moral agent (Habermas, 1996). It follows that procedural justice is not only instrumental in the efficiency of governance but a key feature of the moral structure of democratic legitimacy.

Normative Interpretation: Compliance or Moral Community?

These empirical results pose a more philosophical question: what is the nature of the social order generated by procedural justice? Does it merely extract compliance, or does it build a common moral identity, a sense of political community through recognition and co-invention of norms? On the one hand, insofar as the model developed by Tyler focuses on instrumental trust, that is, a type of compliance founded on perceived legitimacy, critics suggest that this minimizes justice to merely the psychological gratification. In Kantian or Honnethian terms, justice is aimed, at least in part, to declare individuals as worthy of equal moral respect as moral agents who are, or aim to be, in control of their own lives. Properly conceived, procedural justice should be even more than a technology of governance, but also a practice of moral inclusion. It is in this sense that Habermas (1996) insists on the interdependence of legality and legitimacy: laws are valid not because they are enacted but because they emerge from discursive procedures open to all affected parties. Similarly, Young (2002) argues for a deliberative democracy that centers inclusion, difference, and narrative in public reasoning. In this way, procedural justice is not just an instrumental part of moral community, a tool used to achieve behavioral outcomes. It creates confidence not only in institutions, but in other citizens as joint actors in a common normative order.

The relationships between institutional trust and procedural justice and democratic participation are not only the matter of an empirical study; it is more a philosophical question of the terms of political legitimacy and human value. The fact that normative theorists have long insisted on was confirmed empirically: Using just procedures does not only lead to better results but also validates the moral status of those who engage in them. Although fraught with insecurity, procedures of fairness can provide a teeth-edge, and crucial stabilization to a reestablishment of trust in societies built on polarization, exclusion, and epistemic injustice. However, it should not be conceived in terms of a technocratic neutrality but in terms of a normative engagement with recognition, dialogue, and co-authorship. The issue, it follows, is how to devise institutions that not only consider but execute justice in an inclusive, transparent, participatory manner, this in turn creating a community of equals not so much governed as morally bound by processes of justice.

Global South Perspectives: Justice and Well-Being in Development Contexts

The recent empirical attempts to quantify well-being and justice, such as the Human Development Index, OECD Better Life Index, and so on, frequently assume cross-cultural universality of typically Western normative standards. However, the epistemic authority of such metrics has come under fire by scholars of postcolonial theory, critical development studies, and Southern epistemologies. Their critiques focus on how dominant models of development and well-being often exclude, distort, or instrumentalize the values, aspirations, and lived realities of populations in the Global South (Santos, 2014; Nussbaum, 2012).

Critiques of Western Metrics: Epistemological and Ethical Limits

GDP, HDI, and life satisfaction indexes are only descriptive metrics; indeed, they are normative measures, encoding particular expectations about how to live well. As Boaventura de Sousa Santos (2014) argues, these tools are embedded within an "abyssal line" that separates Western knowledge from subaltern epistemologies. This leads to epistemic colonialism, in the sense that Southern ideas of justice and well-being as rooted in the collectivity of autonomy, ecological sustainability, and spiritual belonging become either invisible or unintelligible in the dominant epistemologies. The capabilities approach as developed by Martha Nussbaum can be considered as partly responsive to this criticism, as it focuses on plurality, agency, and human dignity. However, even Nussbaum has been criticized for proposing a "universal list" of capabilities that, while normatively motivated, may risk epistemic imposition when applied without adequate contextual adaptation (Robeyns, 2005). It is not setting aside the comparability issue but decolonizing the standards through which well-being is evaluated and justice is operational. In addition, standardized indicators may tend to promote simplicity at the expense of input that is easily measurable over qualitative, communal, or narratively enmeshed value. This has culminated into development interventions, which despite their numerical success do not accommodate the structural, cultural, and spiritual aspects of injustice. As an example, the opening of schools or clinics could increase HDI scores without giving respect to indigenous languages or customary laws, and the contradiction between successful instrumentalism and cultural appreciation is easily seen.

Participatory Action Research and Local Conceptions of Justice

The tradition of Participatory Action Research (PAR) offers one of the most promising answers to these limitations. Basing its philosophy on emancipatory practice by Paulo Freire and pushed a step further by feminist and postcolonial perspectives, PAR asks: How can we create knowledge alongside communities that are being marginalized, rather than mining data out of them. In development contexts, this means engaging local actors not as beneficiaries but as epistemic agents capable of articulating their own visions of justice and well-being. For instance, participatory poverty assessments conducted by the World Bank in the 1990s and 2000s revealed that communities often defined well-being not in terms of income but in terms of dignity, belonging, and secure relationships (Narayan et al., 2010). Justice was defined in most African and South Asian settings as being able to live without raiding or fighting, to be honored by others in the society and community, to use of the common resources without shame or fear, something that is not captured in the generally accepted indicators. These participatory processes have also shown that outcome equity is less appreciated than fair treatment of people, viz., a sense of being heard, included, and recognized. This realization reminds the superiority of systems of distribution and facilitates the transition to the version of justice that is recognitional and relational and whose support is expressed by such theorists as Nancy Fraser and Iris Marion Young.

In South Africa, India, and Brazil, land reform has become the main point of focus of the justice struggles with the contests seeing the communitarian right to use and stewardship of land opposed with the legalistic, property rights concept of justice. Empirical studies have shown that land redistribution programs are most effective when they incorporate local norms of fairness and collective ownership, rather than imposing top-down allocation schemes (Borras & Franco, 2010). In the case of India, for instance, the Ekta Parishad movement has introduced a focus on land rights not just as a resource problem, but as one of social dignity and cultural life, or even of survival: especially the Adivasi and Dalit populations. In this case, justice is not individualizing titling but is achieved at the collective right and relational land ethics based on ancestral belonging.

Gender Equity and Justice as Empowerment

The maintenance of the justice-as-equality perspectives towards gender-specific development programs is stipulated in the propagation of equal access to teaching, medical and labor markets. This is crucial, even though in the case of gendered injustice, it might not be attentive to cultural and affective features of the phenomenon. For instance, research on women's self-help groups in Bangladesh and Kerala has shown that empowerment is experienced not only as material independence but as recognition of voice, agency, and relational transformation (Kabeer, 1999). Further feminists and women in most settings have created a new definition of justice by focusing on the intra-household command in terms of respect and decision-making, as well as solidarity in communities, which is now challenging individualistic assumptions possessed by most liberal conceptions of development. The redefinitions require intersectional and contextualized measures, i.e., those which point to the lived realities of oppression and emancipation.

This has been the case in Latin America and Oceania, where indigenous peoples have fought and found justice not by assimilating in the quest of integration into state systems but by recognizing autonomous governance, traditional law, and epistemological sovereignty. The Zapatista insurgency in Mexico, by contrast, defines justice not as the state provision of welfare but, rather, as governing with direction and obeying the commands of the governed; a two-way, noncentered political, relational control based in native cosmo-theologies. Empirical studies have shown that such models, though resistant to standard evaluation metrics, contribute to higher subjective well-being, lower violence, and stronger ecological stewardship. The task consists in the attempt to quantify these results without depriving them of their ontological support, which would demand methodological imagination and epistemic modesty.

The Ethical Imperative of Epistemic Justice

Underlying these empirical and normative critiques is the concept of epistemic justice, which concerns the fair distribution of epistemic authority, recognition, and intelligibility (Fricker, 2007). Epistemic injustice occurs in development settings in the form of exclusion of the local knowledge systems in decision-making, downplaying of the knowledge systems as unscientific, and the knowledge systems being appropriated without giving the people concerned. As Santos (2014) puts it, what is needed is not merely more data but an "ecology of knowledges," a pluralist epistemology that values the cognitive diversity of cultures, traditions, and lifeworlds. This is not relativism but reflexive universality, in which universality is created in encounters with the specific in dialogue. Epistemic justice also entails methodological reflexivity. It reminds scholars and policy-makers to ask what is it which is measured, as well as who determines what counts as knowledge, whose voices are listened to, and whose lifeworlds become made visible or invisible. It calls to leave extractive empiricism behind and explore co-creative, dialogical ways of asking and inquiring.

The concepts of justice in the Global South cannot be reduced to a numerical measure based upon liberal individualism, secular-rationalist, or capitalist development as the standard by which justice is measured. Neither can well-being be rendered comprehensively by statistical proxies lacking context, meaning, and voice. It is not and ought not to abandon measurement, but rather one should take a new look at it as a political and moral process, balancing the variety of justice claims, and the reliability of varying modes of knowledge. Global South is not adding an add-on but constituting and correcting. It entails a reconsideration of development as a process not of transferring norms and resources north-way south, but of ethical learning and epistemic co-creation between teaching and learning. It is only in this manner that justice can be made empirically apparent without erasing epistemologically those who do it differently.

Capabilities, Functionings, and Multidimensional Well-Being

The Capability Approach, primarily developed by Amartya Sen (1999) and extended by Martha Nussbaum (2012), marks a paradigmatic shift in how well-being, justice, and development are conceptualized and measured. By dismissing welfarist measures such as utility or income as a proxy to flourishing, the capability framework brings to the fore what people can actually become and do: what are in fact their freedoms or opportunities to enjoy a valued way of living. The revolution of abandoning pointlessness against prospects, products against what products can do, has been deep-rooted both in the normative theory and in the practice.

Operationalizing Capabilities: HDI, IHDI, and OPHI Indices

The renunciation of the open-ended and plural space of capabilities in favor of fixed metrics was even hesitated in by Sen himself. Nevertheless the pressure to test policy introduced pragmatism. The Human Development Index (HDI), introduced by the UNDP in 1990, represented a seminal step away from GDP-centric metrics. It used a composite index of health (life expectancy), education (mean and expected years of schooling), and income (GNI per capita) to reflect basic functionings necessary for a life of dignity. Recognizing the limitations of the HDI in masking inequality, the inequality-adjusted HDI (IHDI) was introduced in 2010. It penalizes countries for disparities across the three dimensions. The achievement of functioning, as measured by both indices, remains narrow when it comes to paying attention to agency, freedom, and choice, the main pillars of the Capability Approach. To address these concerns, the Oxford Poverty and Human Development Initiative (OPHI), led by Sabina Alkire, developed the Multidimensional Poverty Index (MPI). It is a variant of the Alkire-Foster methodology that measures deprivation on 10 indicators in health, education, and living standards and can be decomposed by subgroups of the population and dimension-wise intensity (Alkire & Foster, 2011). Although MPI continues to only be a functions-based indicator, OPHI has started some work on agency-based indicators, such as subjective indicators of powers of control and empowerment, voice, and participation. However, the summarization of such deep descriptions of normative implications into veritable empirical evidence is a philosophical and scientific dilemma.

Household and Individual-Level Capability Data

The use of household-level data was one of the major flaws of early capability measures because it tended to mask intra-household inequalities, especially between women and men and generational issues as well. In response to that, there have been calls in the literature to look at collective-level assessments of capability, which disaggregate education, nutrition, employment, and autonomy.

For example, Kuklys (2005) and Robeyns (2006) emphasize the need to move from aggregate welfare economics to microlevel, person-sensitive analysis that captures differences in conversion factors—i.e., the personal, social, and environmental conditions that mediate the transformation of resources into capabilities. It is of particular relevance to marginalized groups that might have equal access to the same collection of resources, but unequal capability of harnessing them through discrimination and social norms.

Recent surveys such as the India Human Development Survey (IHDS) and Demographic and Health Surveys (DHS) in Sub-Saharan Africa have begun to incorporate such disaggregated data, enabling fine-grained analysis of functionings such as bodily integrity, freedom of movement, decision-making power, and access to social support.

Disparities in Capability Distribution: Gender, Caste, and Region

The basic difference in the distribution of capabilities is one of the most important empirical phenomena, although evidence of meaningful expansion of basic services has improved, the situation has been most notable in India and Sub-Saharan Africa. Nations exhibit gendered shortcomings with respect to education, health, and freedom of movement, which can be highly entrenched and patriarchal in nature, as opposed to a shortage on resources, per se. Women in India, like their counterparts in other parts of the world, have fewer chances compared to their male counterparts to take part in decision-making at the household level, access formal employment, as well as have the freedom to move around, which are critical aspects of agency. Caste also plays a significant role: Dalit and Adivasi communities consistently report lower levels of health, education, and housing, reflecting structural constraints that inhibit capability expansion. Disparity of the region is in turn augmented by conflict, vulnerability of ecology, and colonial extractivism in Sub-Saharan Africa. The Multidimensional Poverty Index disaggregations and Afrobarometer surveys show how disadvantage is exerted in intersecting forms, such as gender, geography, and ethnicity, which can translate into capability deprivation, despite the national averages indicating progress. These empirical facts contribute to the argument to have intersectional capability analysis, where justice is not assessed upon average realization but worst-off, which goes in line with Rawlsian and Senian requirements to prioritize the worst-off.

Conceptual Tensions: Aggregation, Commensurability, and Reification

Although multidimensional indices have helped move the empirical study of well-being forward, they create some form of philosophical tensions. Of utmost concern among them is what we call the problem of aggregation: how can different and qualitatively distinct capabilities, such as political freedom, bodily health, emotional well-being, and capacity to express oneself creatively, be added together into one single index? Sen (1999) resisted endorsing a fixed list or weighted aggregation, preferring a deliberative-democratic approach where different societies articulate their own priorities. In contrast, Nussbaum (2012) proposed a universal list of central capabilities, arguing that certain entitlements are preconditions for any life worthy of dignity. On the one hand, her approach is admirable in its normative clarity only at the cost of crucially essentializing form of human flourishing and thus limiting the openness and pluralism of the Sen model it glorifies.

Further, the process of quantification also has the potential to reify capabilities themselves, and turn an ethically charged term such as dignity or freedom into technocratic data, however, such translation can obscure causal pathways and ethical meanings, producing a "thin or weak" conception of well-being divorced from lived experience. Measurement is not the issue here but on overconfidence in indicators and disregard of the qualitative, contextual, and narrative aspects of human flourishing. Capsules are in danger of being used as an instrument of bureaucratic government, as opposed to an instrument of emancipatory transfiguration, without philosophical reflexivity. The Capability Approach is still one of the most philosophically advanced and empirically conducive methods of connecting justice and well-being. It has made it possible to rethink about poverty, inequality, and development, and has shifted beyond income to look at the real freedoms enjoyed by people. However, its operationalization causes not only conceptual, but also practical, dilemmas: how to focus the normative depth and the empirical clarity, how not to lose the plurality through relativism, and how to make certain that indicators are used as instruments of human goals, but not the means of institutional control.

In the capability measures of justice, one has to be considerate of what is measured and how it is represented, as well as whose priorities inform the assessment. Thereby, the approach reaffirms the value of philosophy in the context of empirical work, not as an abstract idealism but as a critical, normative, and interpretive practice that is fundamentally needed to construct meaningful work in the study of meaningful social measurement.

Justice Metrics and Policy Impact Evaluation

The possibility of testing empirically justice via policy intervention is both a technical problem and a huge philosophical issue. With modern forms of governance more willing and able to embrace evidence-based policy-making, the application of justice-based metrics, including equality of access measures, affirmative inclusion, and empowerment indices, has gained traction. However, the process of normalization of normative ideals into measured achievement causes serious doubts on credibility of justice as both moral and political construct. Using the illustrations of such examples as conditional cash transfers, legal aids, and community-based justice frameworks and universal education schemes, it elaborates how the mechanisms of justice are getting absorbed into the supply apparatus of the state. Lastly, it discusses the philosophical dilemma between policy and moral aftermath as to whether empirical performance is equivalent with normative propriety.

Evaluating Redistributive, Affirmative, and Empowerment Policies

The justice policy review has recently received a center of attention in growth economics, social welfare state governance, and politically human rights-based policy-making. The judgments that are made in these cases usually aim to evaluate the policy efficacy of policies in rectifying inequality, enhancing the agency, and rectifying structural disadvantage. Notably, these appraisal frameworks leave behind the limited measurement of cost–benefit and embrace multidimensional measures of justice such as access, participation, dignity, and capability. Redistributive policies, such as Conditional Cash Transfer (CCT) programs in Latin America (e.g., Bolsa Família in Brazil, Oportunidades in Mexico), are evaluated not only in terms of poverty reduction but in relation to intergenerational equity, gender empowerment, and access to services. They usually relate to such indicators as school attendance, health checks, nutrition results, and the implicit assertion that these latter encode advances in justice as fairness in general.

The indicators of inclusion have been employed in measuring the affirmative action policies, mostly in India, South Africa, and the USA in education, employment, and political representation. These evaluations raise questions about distributive justice, but also about recognition, historical redress, and the deconstruction of entrenched hierarchies. Programs like legal literacy, community courts, and decentralized participatory budgeting are all potential types of empowerment programs that frequently utilize qualitative measures, such as the perceived legal efficacy, self-reported dignity, and community voice. These measures point at justice as a means to improve agency in addition to being a resource disposition.

In both of these areas, justice metrics are characterized as descriptive and aspirational: they are aimed less at describing the actual social reality but rather at presenting an ideal view of what should be done.

Conditional Cash Transfers (CCTs)

The paradigmatic example of such a metric-based assessment of justice-enhancing policy is Bolsa Famiglia and similar programs. Whereas the earlier forms of assessment would involve the parameter of income poverty, the more recent forms include use of gender-sensitive indicators, including more maternal authority, health care access of even daughters, and reduced child labor. Critics however claim that these assessments run the risk of instrumentalizing justice, but act more on behavioral conformity (e.g., sending children to school) than on structural injustices (e.g., inadequate quality of schooling, caste discrimination). The entitlement to trade benefit to practical functioning lacks a balance and is contextual. Plural legal systems have measured community courts and paralegal programs with the following indicators: the speed of resolving a case, the satisfaction of the individual using the community courts and reliance on the paralegal program, and the perceived fairness. Such measures of justice are meant to go beyond formal legality and count substantive access to justice. However, power, cultural pluralism, and moral authority tend to be ignored when translation of complex, relational justice experiences are translated into standardized indicators. The nature of what constitutes a resolution can vary in different communities, namely, in places where traditional law, religious reconciliation, and family are a part of justice definition. Indicators of education justice may incorporate enrollment figures, literacy achievements, and utilization of instructional staff. However, although such metrics may be considered as the indicators of improvement, they tend to ignore more qualitative outcomes of educational justice: the creation of critical agency, the celebration of linguistic diversity, and the embrace of marginalized pasts. Empirical judgments should thus contain narrative, experiential and culturally embedded clues of what should be seen as equitable learning.

Policy Feedback Loops: When Indicators Reshape Governance

One can distinguish the fact that justice measures are part of a policy feedback loop. Indicators do not merely reflect governance priorities, they reshape them. As soon as justice measures are institutionalized in performance systems, funding mechanisms, or international rankings, they can organize bureaucratic conduct and citizen anticipations. For example, India's Right to Education Act created legal entitlements tied to measurable standards (e.g., teacher–student ratios), compelling state governments to reallocate resources and reform administrative practices. Likewise, the World Bank Justice for the Poor project placed a greater focus on the indicators of local-level empowerment, showing an impact on national legal aid plans in recent examples where Indonesia and Sierra Leone changed focus.

These feedback loops highlight the performative capacity of metrics: they change how people reason publicly about justice, economically induce improvement, and change what institutions deem important. However, they also introduce a risk of being captured by the metrics, i.e., meeting indicator controls replacing meeting justice itself.

Philosophical Critique: Are Outcomes a Proxy for Justification?

There is still a major philosophic question, which lies at the core of it all, can empirical results serve as the proxy of moral justification? Does the fact that a policy is able to produce desirable outcomes in any way render it just? From a deontological perspective, this conflation is deeply problematic. Justice, in the meaning given by Kant, involves behavior that respects the moral freedom of individuals but does not involve behaviors that are useful. Even when the policy passes on indicators, it is the literacy achieved by coercion or humiliation that can get it to fall the moral test of dignity. Similarly, Rawlsian liberalism has prioritized specifically procedural fairness and public reason as conditions of justice, along with results. The indicators which count the consequences only, only risk to neglect the issues of consent, deliberation, and the legitimacy.

Moreover, Amartya Sen (2009) cautions against transcendental institutionalism, the idea that a perfectly just institution can be designed in abstraction from comparative real-world analysis. On the one hand, he does insist on empirical assessment, but on the other, he cautions against outputs as being the sole termination of the ethical meaning of justice. The interpretation of them should be within the context of capabilities, freedoms, and agency. Therefore, the measure of justice should be incorporated within the framework of philosophical thought differentiating between means and ends, procedural and substantive, instrumental and intrinsic values. Instruments of justice may be one of the most important instruments of ethical administration, as they facilitate transparency, responsibility, and publicly accountable deliberation. Yet they cannot substitute for normative reflection. Their validity is rooted not only in the technical accuracy but in the philosophical soundness: do they measure what counts, do they cover whom they should, do they serve whom they purport to liberate. Finally, the assessment of policies in terms of justice is an ethical activity and not a statistical one. It demands critical examination of indicators, reflexivity toward context, and adherence to inclusion. It is only when metrics then are able to strengthen, rather than undermine, the moral purpose of justice in the life of a community.

Methodological Reflections: Limits of Quantification in Capturing Justice

The language of governance, policy evaluation, and international development has now been based on quantification. The modern world of policies is taken over by indicators, indices, and rankings, which determine priorities, resource investments, and the manner in which social progress can be meaningfully measured. However, in the strictest things such as justice, quantification becomes a threat of distortion, reductionism, and reification. This is not an ontological and epistemological problem; it is not merely a technical problem of measurement error. It deals with the very nature of the thing justice is, how to think about it, and whether it could be represented in numeric terms in a meaningful manner retaining any moral core. There is a recent literature across philosophy, political theory, and the social sciences that has warned against the risks of subjecting to quantitative frameworks an underlying world that is plural, contentious, and historically defined. Justice is not a value-neutral object of observation, but rather a relation and a series of claims and counter claims, as well as a continuing process of deliberation. Its quantification, is to make decisions, which are explicitly made, which may be implicitly made, about what should be counted, who should count, and how moral goods should be prioritized.

Internal Critique: Sampling Bias, Cultural Translation, and Metric Reification

In the philosophical literature there is one nagging suspicion that we may label normative misfitting: the implication of the empirical instruments and implementations applied to observe and analyze social phenomena cannot grasp the moral core of justice. Three recurring methodological pitfalls illustrate this problem. To begin with the issue of sampling bias is a threat to the issue of representativeness and legitimacy. Surveys that purport to measure public trust, perceptions of fairness, or well-being frequently overrepresent urban, literate, and majority populations, marginalizing voices that are structurally silenced (Smith, 2012). Jurisdiction most sensitive to injustice, the countryside, linguistic minority, and undocumented migrants, often remain out of the datasets upon which justice claims are extrapolated. This process of exclusion reinvigorates injustice in the very measure in which injustice is built into epistemic inequality using the infrastructure of empirical research.

Second, cultural translation presents a serious epistemological challenge. Relatively little attention is paid in most of the dominant justice indicators that are designed in the Global North and offered at the international level without considering the semantic equivalence or contextual specificity. The meanings of concepts like autonomy, fairness, or empowerment could be radically different across the cultural fields. In the contexts where more communitarian ethics apply (e.g., in the societies of Asia or Africa), the concept of autonomy may not be interpreted more as self-determination but rather as a connection one has in a network of mutual duties. Without careful interpretive work, applying liberal-individualist indicators across all societies risks producing not only misleading comparisons but also forms of epistemic imperialism (Sen, 2004).

Third, Metric reification (i.e., treating the indicators of social constructions as ontologically real) has long been criticized in the philosophy of social science. Ian Hacking (1990) famously warned of the "looping effects" of classifications, whereby the categories we create feed back into the social realities they are meant to capture. In justice, this implies that measuring itself may change the behavior of people, the practice of their institutions, and even policy agendas. The indicators develop to be ends in themselves that people can strive to achieve, and not means of obtaining moral goals. As time goes on, a reduction of the richness and ambiguity of lived experiences of justice are lost as their attention is narrowed to what can be counted. All these critiques point to the fact that methodological humility and epistemic reflexivity are known to be necessary. Quantitative measures do not intrinsically have something wrong with them, however; in cases where they seek to be portrayed as the sole contributing factors toward justice, they may give an illusion of impartiality and fulfillment.

Mixed Methods as an Epistemic Imperative

This is not to say that it is true that statistics only allow a qualitative approach to fill in those gaps, but that justice is a lived, narrated, and disputed experience, and therefore has multiple epistemic perspectives. Narrative inquiry is a means of tapping justice as moral experience instead of the ethical state of affairs. By allowing individuals and communities to tell their own stories, researchers can illuminate dimensions of injustice, such as humiliation, disrespect, or invisibility—that rarely register in aggregate data (Polkinghorne, 1988). What the testimonies of survivors, through displacement, violence (caste based), or political repression feign is that justice is in large part not only a matter of possession of material but of recognition and expression. Ethnographic methods base justice on the daily realities of the worlds of ethics. The deeply immersive fieldwork experience can reveal both the relations between legal norms, social practices, and moral expectations and how those interactions can be contradictory. Ethnography has been particularly effective in revealing non-liberal conceptions of justice, such as collectivist, relational, and spiritual dimensions that are absent from liberal-individualist frameworks (Das, 2007).

Participatory surveys go further to reaching the end user by viewing the participant as an epistemic partner (rather than a data point). Drawing on Paulo Freire's (1970) pedagogy of the oppressed and building on methods such as participatory rural appraisal (PRA), these approaches invite communities to define what justice means to them, identify relevant indicators, and co-analyze results. These are ways of democratizing research, protecting against epistemic exclusions of the traditional survey research. In keeping with the positivist view of value-neutral measurement, when used strictly, mixed methods overcome the weaknesses of quantitative tunnels to go far beyond complementing them; they actually attack the positivist dream of value-neutral measurement by demonstrating that all measurement is value-laden.

Value Pluralism and the Problem of Incommensurability

More than technical improvements are needed; however, there is a more philosophical dilemma, the problem of incommensurability. Isaiah Berlin (1969) argued that human values are often plural, irreducible, and sometimes in conflict. When trying to reduce all these disparate moral goods into one-dimensional numerical index, there is danger of normative violence, i.e., the just moral distinctions are swept away in the name of a standardized index. A case in point: African communitarian customs, e.g., ubuntu, that focus on harmony in relationships, embeddedness in the social world, and being connected with ancestors. These values might not and need not fall cleanly along liberal directions of procedural fairness, or individual rights, but they present internally consistent and highly matched moral visions of justice. An index that disregards such conventions is subject to misrepresentation as well as marginalization morally. Value pluralism is realized in incompatible claims to justice in rival systems of meritocracy and redistribution, recognition and neutrality, restorative and retributive justice even within one common society. The application of a unified assessment scheme in these situations is to take positions on still undecided ethical controversies. This is not to say cross-cultural or cross-group comparison is an impossibility but that in doing so one needs a sensitivity to a moral conflict and a readiness to accept that some tensions will go unresolved. Indicators should be designed to reflect, not overwrite, moral diversity.

Normative Guidance Without Instrumentalization

All this brings one more question: what can be an empirical study of justice that will not instrumentalize justice, yet will still be normatively oriented? How then do we invoke data in the service of exposing injustice without reifying justice into data? One possible answer comes from Amartya Sen's (2009) conception of public reasoning. Sen does not believe in a transcendental, fully fleshed out account of theories of justice, but believes in comparative assessments based on open, inclusive, deliberation. Here indicators cannot be considered as unconditional measures; they weigh as heuristics indicators, stimuli to speak, criticize, and learn morally. Nancy Fraser's (2009) theory of participatory parity offers a complementary perspective. In the case of Fraser, justice needs social conditions where members of a society can relate as equals. In this perspective indicators are envisaged not just to measure the results but to multiply democratic capabilities and challenge structural exclusions (Land & Michalos, 2018).

By all this, these structures suggest that the activity of empirical justice research ought to take the form of some sort of critical-constructive ethos: critical in its sensibility to the power, contingency and exclusion; constructive in its obedience to constrainment of knowledge, inclusion and disentanglement. Moral goals should not serve as indicators.

The failure of quantification to seize justice is not, after all, statistical in nature, but ontic, epistemic, and ethical. Justice is not anything that we can count, but what we count, and how we count it, forms the way the governing structure is made up morally. A just methodology is that methodology that acknowledges complexity, hears other voices, adopts plural values, and opposes domination. It quantifies without conquering, symbolizes without scaling back, and leaves open the possibility that not all truths about justice may be susceptible to any sort of numerization at all. To go on, ethical empiricism is needed: a way of inquiry that would bring normative reflection and the empirical study into a collaborative dialogue. Numbers in such an approach speak but so will stories, silences, and struggles. Justice is not only enlightened by statistical correlations but by the personal experiences of the persons whose voice too frequently is not heard. It is only through the dynamic tension between these qualitative and quantitative aspects of rigor, richness, openness, and depth that the inquiry of empirical justice research can escape the twin dangers of technocracy and relativism. Here is where the prospect of a morally informed, methodologically self-reflexive, and politically responsible empiricism can be shaped.

Concluding Summary

The closing of this chapter reiterates a main philosophical argument: empirical investigation is not, and in any case should not, be the exclusive enslavement of predictive truth-claims. Instead, within the terms of its normative enshrinement and reflexive constitution, it makes a formidable medium of moral reflection, able to expose the latent forms of injustice, shed light upon the lived experiences of exclusion, and stimulate popular deliberation to the question of what justice demands. This perspective criticizes the positivism understanding of truth in its epistemology by affirming the empirical data is posed as unique, situational-neutral, and absolute facts. As Hilary Putnam (2002) and Amartya Sen (2009) have argued, fact and value are not dichotomous domains but interdependent aspects of moral reasoning. The entire empirical indicators serve their epistemic role as a normative only in a context of being able to be relevant to the real world and any ethical judgments seeking to be at all in touch with the real world should have an empirical basis. The empirical work in the justice situation can only be viewed as a kind of epistemic action that is on the borderline between the philosophy of criticism and the policy.

Empirical studies are able to bring out the pattern of structural injustice, which abstract moral theory alone may miss especially when used critically and ethically. An example would be the information on gender health inequality, or racialized educational enter exclusion, or inequalities in regions of capability comes in handy in showing to us how systemic the phenomenon of deprivation is, not the individual manifestations. Raw data on the excess killings of Dalit women in India when compared to other Indian women, or the proliferation of Black young people filtered into the US school-to-prison pipeline, go beyond a description of social facts. They validate the embodied experiences of injustice, bringing them into the sphere of public discourse and moral deliberation where they cannot be dismissed as anecdotal or exceptional (Fraser, 2009; Crenshaw, 1989). Data, in turn, themselves may serve as instruments of what Nancy Fraser refers to as participatory parity, the desirable framework in which everyone can participate in social cooperation on equal terms. To describe who is prohibited to speak, to make life undefined is the best empirical research to undertake in the coterminous annihilation of erasure and assert dignity of living. It has ceased to be only a document of disparities but a prescription to the moral being of a society.

Toward a Normatively Embedded Empiricism

The question, then, does not suppose an answer to the question of whether or not to employ empirical methods, but how to employ them so as to respect the moral complexity of justice. What is required is normatively embedded empiricism, that which is:

- Democratic: Underpinned by discussion and popular involvement as opposed to technocratic fiat, such that the things and means of measure are answerable to the subject in whose name and behalf they are involved.
- Plural: It is open to the moral grammars and the cultural understandings of justice, avoiding the temptation to impose a single evaluative framework in all contexts.
- Reflexive: Criticism of its own epistemic biases, exclusions, and structural limitations and is always questioning the conditions under which it gets its knowledge.

Such an approach resonates with Boaventura de Sousa Santos's (2014) call for "epistemologies of the South," which demand the democratization and decolonization of knowledge production. It also aligns with Elizabeth Anderson's (2010) vision of "democratic equality," in which research is accountable to affected communities, not merely to the institutions or funders who commission it. Indicators and statistics taken in this frame are not etalons of investigation but rather beginning of polemic and open deliberations. They are prescribers to group discussions based around the central question: What sort of society are we building and whom? The technologization of justice is challenged through normative entrenched empiricism that maintains empiricism as tentative and dialogical, but not as authoritative and definitive.

Empiricism as Ethical Praxis: A Philosophical Reframing

As this chapter eventually develops, the very notion of empiricism is being put in a new frame, that is, no longer as a science of measuring, but as a moral practice of justice. This sort of reframing places empirical work as a mediator between the moral theory and the reality of the lived life and gives each the power to check the other. This picture of measuring well-being, capability, and justice is not one of encapsulating timeless reality in numbers. It is concerned with the pursuit of common space of reason-giving where claims could be articulated and challenged and transformed. This process is deeply Aristotelian, privileging *phronesis* (practical wisdom) over episteme (theoretical knowledge) as the most appropriate mode of judgment in contexts where value pluralism, uncertainty, and contestation are inevitable. In addition, one that is grounded in normativity is an empiricism that repulses the reduction of justice to bureaucratic administrative convenience or procedure. It retains justice under the concept regulative ideal like the ideal orientation in measurement as opposed to what has to be grasped. This is important because as soon as justice is made into an object that can be evaluated with certainty it faces the risk of being marginalized in favor of institutions instead of institutionalizing it.

Looking Ahead: From Philosophy to Policy Practice

The conclusion serves as pretext to Chap. 6 that will cover the application of the normative-empirical approach elaborated in this work onto three strategic spheres, namely, health, education, and environmental policy. Of both, there is an immediate and argued relationship between justice and well-being, so they are rich places to consider how metrics are applied, interpreted, and manipulated in institutional practice. In the realm of public health, we will explore how indicators can either obscure or reveal what Miranda Fricker (2007) calls "epistemic injustice, " the exclusion of certain groups from the capacity to contribute to shared understandings of their own needs. The study of education policy, on the contrary, will be discussed with the opposition between the access development and cultural recognition by focusing on the aspect that justice owes more than equal enrolment numbers. Environmental policy will bring into focus intergenerational and ecological justice, raising questions about how current metrics capture (or fail to capture) long-term obligations to future persons and nonhuman life. In all these spheres we are faced with the same question: do our mediating empirical means widen our moral perception or do they narrow it? The model described in this chapter would lead to a response that it cannot only be answered based on methodological vigor, but on the normative commitment too. An ethically constituted form of empirical inquiry is not merely an accessory to the cause of justice, but it is a tool of necessity of public reasoning. It is concerned not to tell us what we should value, but to enable us, in more thoughtful and accessible ways, to make out what is at stake when our deliberations turn upon values. The fact that empirical work brings the invisible to visibility and the excluded to view can make an important transformative contribution to democratic life. However, such a transformational potential shall be achieved just in case empirical research does not abandon the principles of democratic participation, moral pluralism, and epistemic reflexivity. Devoid of such promises, measurement can very easily turn into an instrument of subjugation instead of emancipation. At least with them it can come to form part of a sustained practice of justice, a project that must not only join the analytic precision of philosophy and the evidentiary power of social science but must also welcome into its vision a more equal, more dignified, more humane society.

References

Alkire, S., & Foster, J. (2011). Counting and multidimensional poverty measurement. *Journal of Public Economics, 95*(7–8), 476–487.

Anderson, E. (1995). *Value in ethics and economics*. Harvard University Press.

Anderson, E. (1999). What is the point of equality? *Ethics, 109*(2), 287–337.

Anderson, E. (2010). *The imperative of integration*. Princeton University Press.

Bartky, S. L. (1990). *Femininity and domination: Studies in the phenomenology of oppression*. Routledge.

Berlin, I. (1969). *Four essays on liberty*. Oxford University Press.

Borras, S. M., & Franco, J. C. (2010). Contemporary discourses and contestations around pro-poor land policies and land governance. *Journal of Agrarian Change, 10*(1), 1–32.

Butler, J. (2004). *Undoing Gender*. Routledge.

Cartwright, N. (2007). *Hunting causes and using them: Approaches in philosophy and economics*. Cambridge University Press.

Christopher, J. C. (1999). Situating psychological well-being: Exploring the cultural roots of its theory and research. *Journal of Counseling & Development, 77*(2), 141–152.

Crenshaw, K. (1989). Demarginalizing the intersection of race and sex. *University of Chicago Legal Forum, 1989*(1), 139–167.

Das, V. (2007). *Life and words: Violence and the descent into the ordinary*. University of California Press.

Diener, E., Suh, E., Lucas, R., & Smith, H. (1999). Subjective Well-being: Three decades of progress. *Psychological Bulletin, 125*(2), 276–302.

Eisenberger, N. I., Lieberman, M. D., & Williams, K. D. (2003). Does rejection hurt? An fMRI study of social exclusion. *Science, 302*(5643), 290–292.

Esping-Andersen, G. (1990). *The three worlds of welfare capitalism*. Princeton University Press.

Fehr, E., & Gächter, S. (2000). Fairness and retaliation: The economics of reciprocity. *Journal of Economic Perspectives, 14*(3), 159–181.

Folbre, N. (2001). *The invisible heart: Economics and family values*. New Press.

Fraser, N. (2009). *Scales of justice: Reimagining political space in a globalizing world*. Columbia University Press.

Fredrickson, B. L., & Roberts, T. A. (1997). Objectification theory. *Psychology of Women Quarterly, 21*(2), 173–206.

Fricker, M. (2007). *Epistemic injustice: Power and the ethics of knowing*. Oxford University Press.

Gallup. (2023). *Global emotions report*. Gallup, Inc.

Goffman, E. (1963). *Stigma: Notes on the Management of Spoiled Identity*. Prentice-Hall.

Habermas, J. (1996). *Between facts and norms*. MIT Press.

Hacking, I. (1990). *The taming of chance*. Cambridge University Press.

Helliwell, J. F., & Huang, H. (2008). How's your government? International evidence linking good government and well-being. *British Journal of Political Science, 38*(4), 595–619.
Helliwell, J. F., Layard, R., & Sachs, J. (2018). *World happiness report*. Sustainable Development Solutions Network.
Helliwell, J. F., & Putnam, R. D. (2004). The social context of well-being. *Philosophical Transactions of the Royal Society B, 359*(1449), 1435–1446.
Honneth, A. (1995). *The struggle for recognition: The moral grammar of social conflicts*. Polity Press.
Kabeer, N. (1999). Resources, agency, achievements: Reflections on the measurement of women's empowerment. *Development and Change, 30*(3), 435–464.
Kahneman, D., & Deaton, A. (2010). High income improves evaluation of life but not emotional well-being. *Proceedings of the National Academy of Sciences, 107*(38).
Kuklys, W. (2005). *Amartya Sen's capability approach: Theoretical insights and empirical applications*. Springer.
Land, K. C., & Michalos, A. C. (2018). Fifty years after the social indicators movement: Has the promise been fulfilled? *Social Indicators Research, 135*(3), 835–868. https://doi.org/10.1007/s11205-017-1571-y
Link, B. G., & Phelan, J. C. (2001). Conceptualizing Stigma. *Annual Review of Sociology, 27*, 363–385.
Litz, B. T., et al. (2009). Moral injury and moral repair in war veterans. *Clinical Psychology Review, 29*(8), 695–706.
Lynch, J., et al. (2004). Is income inequality a determinant of population health? *The Milbank Quarterly, 82*(1), 5–99.
Michalos, A. C., & Hatch, P. M. (2020). Good societies, financial inequality and secrecy, and a good life: From Aristotle to Piketty. *Applied Research in Quality of Life, 15*(3), 1005–1054. https://doi.org/10.1007/s11482-019-09717-0
Meyer, I. H. (2003). Prejudice, social stress, and mental health in lesbian, gay, and bisexual populations. *Psychological Bulletin, 129*(5), 674–697.
Narayan, D., Patel, R., Schafft, K., Rademacher, A., & Koch-Schulte, S. (2010). *Voices of the poor: Can anyone hear us?* Oxford University Press. for the World Bank.
Nussbaum, M. C. (2012). *Women and human development: The capabilities approach*. Cambridge University Press.
Nussbaum, M. C. (2013). *Creating capabilities: The human development approach*. Harvard University Press.
OECD. (2021a). Income inequality update: Income inequality remains high in the face of the COVID-19 crisis. OECD Publishing.
OECD. (2021b). *Government at a glance*. OECD Publishing.
Polkinghorne, D. E. (1988). *Narrative knowing and the human sciences* (SUNY series in philosophy of the social sciences) (p. 213). State University of New York Press.
Putnam, H. (2002). *The collapse of the fact/value dichotomy and other essays*. Harvard University Press.
Putnam, R. D. (2000). *Bowling alone: The collapse and revival of American Community*. Simon & Schuster.
Rawls, J. (1971). *A theory of justice*. Harvard University Press.
Robeyns, I. (2005). The capability approach: A theoretical survey. *Journal of Human Development, 6*(1), 93–117.
Robeyns, I. (2006). The capability approach in practice. *Journal of Political Philosophy, 14*(3), 351–376.
Ryff, C. D., & Singer, B. (1998). The contours of positive human health. *Psychological Inquiry, 9*(1), 1–28.
Santos, B. d. S. (2014). *Epistemologies of the south: Justice against epistemicide*. Routledge.
Sen, A. (1985). Well-being, agency and freedom: The Dewey lectures 1984. *The Journal of Philosophy, 82*(4), 169–221.

Sen, A. (1999). *Development as freedom*. Oxford University Press.
Sen, A. (2004). How does culture matter? In Rao & Walton (Eds.), *Culture and public action*. Stanford University Press.
Sen, A. (2009). *The idea of justice*. Harvard University Press.
Smith, L. T. (2012). *Decolonizing methodologies: Research and indigenous peoples*. Zed Books.
Tyler, T. R. (2006). *Why people obey the law*. Princeton University Press.
Tyler, T. R., & Blader, S. L. (2003). The group engagement model. *Journal of Personality and Social Psychology, 85*(5), 853–865.
UNDP. (2016). Legal empowerment strategies at the local level.
World Justice Project. (2023). *Rule of law index*.
Young, I. M. (2002). *Inclusion and democracy*. Oxford University Press.

Chapter 6
Justice in Health, Education, and Environmental Policy

Introduction

Justice as historically understood as an abstract philosophical concept must be persistently addressed as a substantive, institutionalized and sectorally personified norm. As Amartya Sen (2009) compellingly argues, the philosophical pursuit of justice gains its moral force not in the construction of ideal institutions but in comparative judgments about lived injustices. In order to philosophize justice in the contemporary context, one must ask what it means to actualize justice sectorally the way it is constructed, blocked, or performed in health care systems, educational systems, and environmental governance. The departure of justice in general to justice in context must personalize a metaphysical abstraction to political and social criticism. While Rawls (1971) remains the architect of justice as fairness in institutional design, contemporary concerns with global justice, identity-based exclusion, and ecological precarity urge a more embedded approach. Ethics of the common good, particularly health, education, and environment, comes into the picture and the theoretical commitments are challenged by the distributive, procedural and recognitional demands.

Public Goods, Political Sites: Health, Education, and the Environment

Health, education, and the environment are not merely instrumental goods but constitutive elements of human flourishing (Nussbaum, 2013). They are both publicly beneficial, in both an economic and moral sense: they are non-excludable, foundational to the development of capabilities, and essential to democratic agency. But they are also locations of distributive unfairness, political conflict, and epistemic

S. K. Maurya, *Exploring Justice as a Social Indicator of Life*, Social Indicators Research Series 92, https://doi.org/10.1007/978-3-032-10812-8_6

contestation. Health cannot be reduced to its biomedical access to include social determinants classified by housing, nutrition, clean water, and systematic discrimination. Justice in health requires attention not only to outcome inequalities but also to institutional responsiveness, cultural respect, and intergenerational equity (Daniels, 2008). Education does not only determine the level of income/productivity, but also the moral and political agency of people. As Elizabeth Anderson (2007) argues, educational justice entails not only access and funding parity but recognition of cultural identity, linguistic diversity, and narratives of belonging. Normative and empirical challenges of environmental justice are some of the most complicated ones. Climate change, biodiversity loss, and toxic exposure reveal how ecological burdens are inequitably distributed, particularly among racialized, Indigenous, and economically marginalized communities (Schlosberg, 2007; Nixon, 2013). The justice that is needed here must have a temporal and spatial imagination that involves nonhuman agents, future generations of existence, as well as interdependence among planets. These domains, while distinct, are normatively entangled. They constitute the institutional infrastructure of justice and the moral supports of the public life.

Why Sectoral Justice Matters: Beyond Aggregative Measures

Broad social indicators, such as the Human Development Index (HDI) or the OECD's Better Life Index, attempt to quantify well-being across dimensions. Nevertheless, they tend to conceal structural circumstances in which life chances are determined. Within that field, sectoral justice analysis enables us to disaggregate well-being into its moral dimensions because we are not simply asking whether people live longer or learn more; we are also asking whether they are treated with dignity, represented in decision-making, and not harmed. This approach also highlights intersectionality and compounding disadvantage. In India, a rural Dalit woman can be exposed to environmental deterioration, school failure, and reproductive health indifference not simply as distinct civic harms, but as intersecting injustices bolstering one another. Without sectoral analysis, such entanglements remain invisible, and policy responses risk being technocratic rather than emancipatory (Fraser, 2009). The overall effect of unfair sectoral outcomes is not simply economic in its impact; it is also to undermine democratically based legitimacy, social solidarity, and public confidence. When access to clean air, quality education, or adequate health care is seen as a privilege rather than a right, the normative foundation of democratic equality is fundamentally undermined (Anderson, 2013).

The Philosophical Challenge: Reconciling Justice Paradigms

One of the major theoretical projects in sectoral justice has been the attempt to harmonize paradigms of distributive, procedural, and recognitional forms of justice. Distributive justice involves equitable mode of distribution of resources, services, and opportunities; it gives rise to the following questions: who gets what and why? This could imply equal access to vaccines in health; equal teacher quality in education; and, in the environment, equal distribution of climate adaptation finance. In procedural justice, the focus is on the equitableness of the decision-making process. It raises the issue of whether health policies have been arrived at through participatory challenges, whether education has been shared or shared out with marginalized communities, or whether Indigenous knowledge systems have been considered during environmental appraisal. Recognitional justice, drawing from Axel Honneth (1995) and Nancy Fraser, focuses on the cultural-symbolic dimensions of justice, how identities are honored or misrecognized. It requires that policies should not only be fairly distributed, but that they respect multiple worldviews, linguistic variety, and shared histories. These dimensions often exist in tension. A distributive measure may reflect equality in test scores and continue to be present in procedural exclusion and cultural alienation in the classrooms. In analogical fashion, the allocation of health resources might be equal, but the medical racism or transphobic norms impair the recognitional and procedural justice. The philosophical inquiry then needs to avoid the approaches of reductive monism but it needs to create integrative systems of multiple justice claims having a dynamic balance. This demands an imperfect, comparative, progressive process that is more aptly called capability perspective and deliberative democratic ethos as opposed to the static theories of perfect justice. Sectoral justice forms the location of the interface between philosophy and governance, and the place of moral commitments refined in the molten rock of policy. Doing justice in health, education, and environmental policy is not just to ensure efficiency or equity in the delivery of the service, it is to create institutions that acknowledge human dignity, participatory agency, and institutions that support the very conditions of life. These domains will be examined throughout this chapter as it delves into how justice is pursued (or where justice is not pursued), or the ways that justice is reimagined in terms of empirical research and metrics of justice and philosophical opinions. The idea is to manifest a plural, critical, ethical-focused familiarity with justice as it is, -and as it may continuing to be -embodied in the material infrastructure of the societal lives.

Justice in Health: Ethics, Access, and Agency

Distributive Justice and the Right to Health

Health care is a morally burdened area that is not just a biological or clinical state but, in many ways, poses the most important questions regarding fairness, equality, and human dignity. The debate about justice in health care does not merely make us question who gets what; it also makes us question such distributions in terms of which normative premises, institutional frameworks, and ethical standards they can be justified. Two prevailing philosophical traditions, such as egalitarianism and sufficientarianism, provide different sets of parameters of addressing the right to health that has policy and practice implications. Egalitarian theories, most notably represented by Norman Daniels (2008), draw from Rawlsian premises to argue that health is a prerequisite for the fair equality of opportunity. According to Daniels, the right to health is neither an exclusive good, but part of his/her ability to pursue life plans on a similar playing field. Based on this view, inequality in access to health care or in health outcomes is injustice in so far as it undermines the capacity of individuals to exercise their capability as the free and equal citizens. To have equal opportunity, it is therefore desirable that the social determinants of health, i.e., income, education, and living conditions also receive attention, in addition to health care delivery. By contrast, sufficientarian theories, influenced by the works of Amartya Sen (2002, 2009), emphasize ensuring that all individuals reach a minimum threshold of health that allows them to achieve basic functioning. It is skills that are important and not equality itself. It is not that it is the uniformity of health outcomes that matters but it is that everyone should be given the possibility to attain substantive freedom and lead the life of dignity. This method is possibly more dynamic, context-specific, and it aims at preventing inadequacies instead of filling all the gaps.

One of the fundamental philosophical contradictions arises between the equality of access and equality of outcomes. The similarity in access to health care facilities does not necessarily mean similar results to be achieved, especially in light of the fact that social determinants of health, say, gender, caste, race, and geography, differ significantly across populations. A Rawlsian egalitarian would be most interested in procedural fairness and the institutional setup that guarantees the acquisition of opportunities whereas a capabilities theorist in the manner of Sen would be keen to emphasize the necessity of justice that is sensitive to the existing disparities in the actual world that put a strain on the conversion of health care into meaningful well-being. As Michael Marmot (2005) has observed, "health inequities are socially produced, systematic in their distribution, and unjust." This implies that health justice theories cannot afford to be institutionally neutral and minimally moral. They are required to deal with the intermeshing of medical systems and their exposure to different social, political, and economic systems of shaping well-being. Without the identification of such, even the most advanced conceptual philosophy models can be sidelined in favor of the disregard of the lived realities of the very people they claim to be serving.

Empirical Evidence and Policy Practices

The philosophical theories of health justice can be imbued with more normative weight and weight of reasonability when they are forced into the light of empirical evidence, that is, the existential realities of health injustice, and the realizations that come out in attempts carried out by governments, communities, and even international agencies. A number of real life cases enlighten both the potential as well as the constraints of institutional commitment to fair health. The United Kingdom's National Health Service (NHS) is perhaps one of the most significant institutional embodiments of health justice. The NHS was established on concepts of universality, comprehensiveness, and equity, which means that the health system addresses health as a social right instead of a marketable commodity. It actualizes a solidaristic ethic by supplying free health care at point of use. The match in terms of all the population however is evident in the form of regional and socioeconomic inequalities in outcomes, and thus institutional design, while important, is not enough to end health disparities altogether (Michalos & Hatch, 2020).

There are gaps in health outcomes caused by social determinants lying beyond the health care system, including housing, nutrition, and education, which are reproducing themselves. Cuba's health care system offers another instructive case. Long-term constraints in economic terms notwithstanding, the country has managed to bring about health indicators as similar to the ones of high-income countries such as low infant mortality and high life expectancy through the system of primary care, community health networks, and preventive medicine. This model questions the premise that equitable health outcomes are only attainable when an economy enjoys a wide range of economic resources, but as demonstrated in the model, political will power, community involvement, and a preventive approach to health strategies can be rewarding on an exceptional scale. Grassroots initiatives such as India's Accredited Social Health Activist (ASHA) program and Ethiopia's Health Extension Program also highlight the potential of decentralized, community-embedded approaches. ICTs in partnership with health initiatives training local women as health workers can reach the rural and marginalized population with access to basic health care, where formal health systems fail to exist and/or are inaccessible. In addition to the enhancement of health statistics, these efforts create empowerment, local control, and community-provider trust.

It is interesting to note that a very visible manifestation of health injustice is the situation of maternal health. According to statistics provided by WHO, UNICEF, and the Guttmacher Institute, the rates of maternal mortality between Indigenous and Black women are remarkably high even in rich countries. Such imbalances are not run-of-the-mill statistical artifacts but rather expression of structural racism, access obstacles, and epistemic neglect in the clinical encounter. The fact that the gaps in question have not been eliminated even in domains with a highly developed health care infrastructure reflects the role of the inherent limitations to access-oriented policies when the underlying causes of these disparities, i.e., bias, discrimination, and cultural competence, have not been addressed. Quantitative variables: the differences in life expectancy, burden of disease, child mortality rates, and geographical accessibility are necessary to develop inequalities mapping. However, they tend to miss the qualitative aspects of injustice, which entail experiences of disrespectful maternity care, a wide range of gender-based violence, or the psychological burden of endemic exclusion. Because of this, deeper evaluations of health justice require the incorporation of statistical measures alongside narrative, ethnographic and participatory measures that reflect lived experience. This is the only way policy can respond fully to moral imperatives, which are inherent in health.

Normative and Methodological Challenges

Although there has been theory and practice advancement, the specific area of health cannot make progress on justice due to the long-standing ethical situations and methodological tensions. Among the most urgent ones is the trade-off between moral urgency and cost effectiveness. Global health funding decisions often rely on measures like Disability-Adjusted Life Years (DALYs) and Quality-Adjusted Life Years (QALYs), which rank interventions by statistical efficiency. While useful for resource allocation, these tools can inadvertently devalue the lives of the elderly, the disabled, or the terminally ill, and can obscure moral priorities such as need, dignity, and relief of suffering (Anand & Hanson, 1997). Epistemic injustice presents another profound challenge. As Miranda Fricker (2007) defines it, epistemic injustice occurs when individuals or groups are wronged specifically in their capacity as knowers. This can be applied to health situations population health survey fails to sub-classify data by the essential indicators of identity, like caste, gender identity, or indigeneity, or the signs and reports of the marginalized patients who release the allegations are negatively constructed by the systems. Indicatively, studies have reported that under-evaluation and treatment of pain experienced by Black patients is a common observation and possibly due to implicit biases, which cannot be fixed merely using quantitative surveillance efforts.

In surges, when faced with short supply of limited resources such as ventilators and ICU beds, triaging protocols needed to be established and this opened a very contentious ethical dilemma: the preferential allocation by age, comorbidity, or by chance of survival? Does saving as many lives as possible always amount to defending the least advantaged? Vaccination equity evolved into a bigger battleground, which saw high-income countries getting early and vast quantities of vaccine stock, to the extent of stockpiling in some cases against need in the face of lower-income countries lagging behind in pulling the vaccine stock. The COVAX initiative did not quite achieve its equity targets, which shows the shortfalls of charity-based approaches in transforming structural inequities. These realities of the age of pandemic compel us to come to grips with the realization that justice in health is not per duck calculus of advantages and harms. It also has to contend with colonial legacies, national self-interest, and structural violence as they define global health relations.

Without the accommodation of such more profound political, historical determinants, we can discover that distributive policies can reinforce existing hierarchies in the spirit of fairness.

To possess a robust understanding of health justice that is beneficial, one must therefore be able to go beyond the technocratic terms of coverage ratio and efficiency scores. It must take note that health is a human potential and a claim to justice. Such a vision would integrate:

- Egalitarian justice in institutional construction, where everyone is given a real chance to be and stay healthy.
- The sufficientarian ensures that no one will languish below the level of functioning essential to a life of dignity.
- Procedural and epistemic justice that ensure involvement and recognition of the marginalized communities in formulation of health policy.
- The global solidarity that provides an alternative to vaccine nationalism and transnational neglect, based on the theories of cooperation and mutual responsibility.

By straddling theory and evidence, ethics and empiricism, local and international demands, another aspect of the cause of justice in health becomes incubated: the pursuit of justice in health is more than just a policy issue; it is a morale test of a society. The health systems that adhere to this type of integration do not just validate the biological survival of the populations they serve, but also the more fundamental state of human flourishing.

Justice in Education: Equality, Recognition, and Human Development

Philosophical Theories of Educational Justice

The quest of justice within the education context cannot be narrowed down to issues of financial distributions, testing, and judging by performance. Instead, it demands long-term commitment with extensive normative absurdness concerning human potential, social equality, and political membership. In this broader understanding, educational justice is interested not just in the distribution of resources but also in their understanding, appreciation, and enabling of individuals in achieving their capabilities. In the philosophical literature there are two predominant paradigms, the equal opportunity and the capability to learn, which present dissimilar but complementary ways of theorizing educational justice.

Equal opportunity theorists, such as John Rawls (1971) and Elizabeth Anderson (2007), argue that justice demands neutralizing the influence of arbitrary social factors, race, class, gender, and other markers of inherited advantage—on life outcomes, including educational attainment. In this light, the education system ought to become a leveling agent whereby different people, with different backgrounds and origins, can compete equally to secure access to advantaged positions within the society. The provision of quality education, equal resource distribution, and equal treatment is the core of this vision. However, critics of the equal opportunity model point out that it presupposes a competitive model of society and does not question the underlying circumstances that are needed to bring out successful learning. The cultural capital state, language identification, and emotional security feeling in the learning environment are not accidentuous remarks about the opportunities of the scholar success but its constituent. When educational justice is stripped of trying to oppose the meritocratic sorting, it can easily become a means of legitimizing such a social hierarchy instead of criticizing it, as Anderson herself recognizes.

In contrast, the capability approach, most prominently developed by Martha Nussbaum (2013) foregrounds what learners are actually able to do and to be. This perspective of justice in education implies more than providing students with an equal opportunity to compete, but the ability of every learner to excel in critical thinking and knowledge, imaginative thinking, and participation in the reasoning life of their community. Flourishing, rather than competitive success, becomes the ultimate goal. Beyond distributive concerns, theorists such as Nancy Fraser (2009) and Iris Marion Young (2022) emphasize that education is also a site of recognition and a medium of democratic inclusion. The systematic degradation of the identities of students, be they racial, linguistic, gendered, or religious, cannot be repaired in its entirety by the amount of access or funding. Recognition-based narratives, in turn, demand that curriculum subject, classroom atmosphere, and teacher–student relationships, are ethical landforms with either justice or misrecognition committed on a daily basis.

From this perspective, civic education assumes a pivotal role. It cannot be simply seen as teaching of political facts, instead, as becoming familiar with standards and procedures of deliberative democracy. Following Amy Gutmann (1999) and Seyla Benhabib (1996), justice requires that education prepare students for mutual respect, critical inquiry, and collective self-rule. Education without such nurture of democratic dispositions is not only likely to be incomplete but unfair, since it will leave future citizens unable to use the skills they have assumed to become valuable participants in the lives of their communities.

Empirical Dimensions and Global Indicators

Even in philosophical areas that are fairly unambiguous there is a gap between translating educational justice into practice involving complexity at the empirical level. Global indicators such as those used by UNESCO, the Human Development Index (HDI), and the Programme for International Student Assessment (PISA) provide quantifiable measures of literacy rates, school attendance, and standardized test performance. These metrics facilitate cross-national comparison and inform policy evaluation. Instead, they are more inclined to remember the contextual richness of local education systems, devalue the difference in culture, and underestimate the noncognitive component of learning. An example is PISA scores, which test the achievement of the 15-year-old population in mathematics, reading, and science. Although these are essential areas, they do not provide much information on the equity of access, linguistic inclusion, or moral and civic development of the education systems. A nation can show very large aggregate numbers but with great inequalities despite lines of caste, ethnicity, or gender, an inequality that statistical averages can mask. Case studies illustrate how these patterns manifest. In India, affirmative action policies such as reservations for Scheduled Castes (SCs), Scheduled Tribes (STs), and Other Backward Classes (OBCs) aim to redress historical educational exclusion. These have widened access especially in higher education although they are disputed. Critics allege that reservations compromise merit, while defenders argue they are still insufficient to address entrenched structural inequalities (Deshpande, 2014). This has led to decades of legal and political controversy in the USA in an effort to assure racial diversity by using affirmative action during university admissions (Fisher v. University of Texas 2016). Another area where the question of justice emerges is language of instruction. The language policy in countries such as South Africa, Nepal, and Canada becomes a debate that is very much related to the subject of recognition and inclusion in a multilingual society. When children are taught in a language foreign to their home environment, they face cognitive hurdles as well as symbolic erasure of their cultural identity (Skutnabb-Kangas, 2013). The problem of linguistic democracy in schooling therefore is not only one concerning that which is educationally effective, but that which is right.

School funding mechanisms further complicate the picture. In America, the funding of schools through local property makes realistic differences between rich and poor school districts drastic. The differences in available funding might become smaller in more centralized systems, like parts of Europe, but inequality is still perpetuated by urban–rural disparities, disconnects in internet access, and the impact of tutoring markets. These patterning structures point out to an educational justice that necessarily needs to be addressed at various levels, reforming the funding, curricular innovations, teacher training, and the community. Finally, the empirical record proves that justice in education cannot be derived only by measures of access or attainment. It should consider the conditions under which learning occurs, the dispositions and structures that confer opportunity, and the way the learners themselves are assigned values as human beings in their schooling conditions.

Methodological and Ethical Reflections

The overlap between philosophical theory and factual observations creates methodological and ethical dilemmas concerning the definition of what constitutes a quality education to be taught and by whom. Western epistemic assumptions are likely to be coded into standardized measures, favoring the knowledge types that are characterized by abstract thinking, quick knowledge production, and easily quantifiable outcomes. These frameworks pose a threat to marginalization of other traditions of knowledge, which are relational, place-based, or spiritually informed. When these perspectives are excluded, education becomes a tool of epistemic domination, legitimizing certain ways of knowing while suppressing others (de Sousa Santos, 2014). This critique has direct implications for curriculum design. Curriculum justice means more than adding a diversity of people, more than bringing a diversity of people to the table; it demands a structural reconsideration of whose history is taught, whose literature is placed on the curriculum, and whose work in science is acknowledged. Feminist scholars such as bell hooks (1994) and Sara Ahmed (2017) have shown how ostensibly neutral pedagogical spaces often reproduce sexism, racism, and heteronormativity, reinforcing rather than dismantling social hierarchies. The query of who actually should and can educate whom is pressing too. The education of marginalized populations is routinely framed as a passive process of receiving, rather than co-constructing, the meaning and substance of education. Decolonial theorists claim that fair education needs to do more than meaningfully incorporating the marginalized learners into the current systems. Instead, it demands a reconstitution of the frameworks themselves (Tuck & Yang, 2012). This movement redefines justice not as access to knowledge that dominates, but as a reclamation and cogeneration of knowledge based on ancestral inheritances, local ways of doing, and embodied knowing. Based on these considerations of method and ethics, the process of pursuing justice in education appears as a multidimensional endeavor. It is distributive, it is nondiscriminatory, there is equitable access to resources and opportunities; it is recognitional, it respects dignity and identity of all learners; and it is participatory, involving communities in structuring and content of education. The element of the just education system as such is therefore that which not only even levels the playing field, but alters the very game, the game which opens up the horizons of what is constituted as knowledge, who is allowed to speak, and what is brought to an end by the knowledge that is directed to the human development and democracies.

Justice and the Environment: Intergenerational and Global Ethics

Environmental Justice as Distributive and Procedural Claim

The environment can no longer be taken as an inert background to human action; an ethical battleground, distributional inequality, and procedural exclusion have become involved. Environmental justice has developed at the very point of understanding and confronting how ecological destruction is disseminated and how it tends to fall upon the socially weakened organization and, conversely, the strong. The pluralist theory of environmental justice by David Schlosberg (2007) represents a significant reconceptualization in that they do not only refer to distributive justice, which is only concerned with who receives what. However, Schlosberg points out, other injustices are generated by the failure to adequately recognize the identities of marginalized communities, and the tendency to lock their voices out of environmental governance. For instance, communities of color in the USA or Dalit populations in India face dramatically increased likelihood of being located near a landfill, a polluting industry, or degraded ecology, with all these disadvantages forcing them to risk health and social stigma, yet lacking appropriate representation in decisions affecting them.

Theories of justice, as articulated by Rawls, beg the question: how a theory of justice developed in the context of closed societies can be modified to respond to the transboundary and intergenerational character of ecological harm? Rawls' astute difference principle, the initially established connection to fellow citizens present at a given time, demands a drastic redefinition in light of the climate debt where the industrialized countries requite remunerations to the Global South due to years of climatic exploitation. It is such obligations that form the essence of the modern demands of climate reparation and in the differentiated obligations of the international agreements such as the Paris Accord.

The ecological debt is a concept that questions the moral neutrality premise of property rights. To the extent that some countries or companies have over the past tapped more than their fair share of ecological resources and in particular carbon space, justice demands a system of historical culpability and redistributive justice (Caney, 2010). These are not questions that can be isolated in the broad social context within which environmental damage transpires. There is a strong intersection between environmental degradation and race, class, gender, and the effects of colonization. This same slow violence of desertification, pollution, and rising sea-levels, as Nixon (2013) makes out eloquently, is most acutely felt by poor, racialized, Indigenous, and formerly colonized people. These groups bear the brunt of environmental degradation and also get systematically locked out of environmental decisions that further entrench practice of procedural unfairness. In this regard, a healthy perception of environmental justice should be pluralistic in its substance and intersectional in its approach. It has to combine distributive justice, recognitional respect, and participatory inclusion with appreciating that harms to ecology are never just ecological, they are always social and political too.

Empirical Studies and Justice Metrics

In order to implement the principles of environmental justice in practice, it is necessary to find an empirical tool to make the spatial, demographic, and historical distributions of harm visible. A series of measures of justice have been formulated to accomplish this, all of which have rather different strong and weak points. The Carbon inequality measures, such as those conducted by Oxfam and the report of Carbon inequality by Chancel and Piketty (2015), show that the richest 10 percent of the world population actually made about half of the total emissions, whereas the poorest 50 percent only made 10 percent of the total emissions. These extreme asymmetries erode utilitarian reasoning in favor of policies guided by environmental growth and provide support to egalitarian or sufficiency policies that put emphasis on satisfying basic needs first before allowing more resource enrichment by the fortunate. The other indicators are concerned with the availability of clean water and air. As an example, such persistent inequalities, both cross-country and between groups in the same country, can be observed in the WHO Air Quality Database. The urban slums, rural perimeters, and Indigenous land usually do not have safe drinking water, experience continuous exposure to hazardous particulate material, including PM2.5, or are forced to live in close contact with harmful waste. These environmental loadings commonly coincide with socioeconomic marginalization, and this increases inequity.

The most renowned of them are the Social Vulnerability Index (SVI) and the Climate Risk Index (CRI), which consider socioeconomic and geographic factors showing how vulnerable populations are likely to find themselves in floods, hurricanes, droughts, and other disasters. The tools are useful in setting directions on adaptation funding, but their assumptions regarding norms such as what constitutes vulnerability, and what communities should adhere to them, are seldom examined critically in an ethical way. The case studies demonstrate that even the environmental policies can be in a way self-perpetuating injustice. In some regions of Global South, the implementation of climate adaptation policies like resettlements or zoning protection schemes has displaced Indigenous communities. These policies, aimed at environmental goals, often prioritize Indigenous communities as disruptors of the environment, rather than recognizing them as preservers of environmental wisdom. The Indigenous-led movement to save the Amazon rainforest and the indigenous resistance at Standing Rock in the USA against the construction of an oil pipeline have indicated that environmental justice cannot be discussed outside of movements to assert sovereignty, identification, and cultural survival.

The development of the term of just energy transitions is testimony to the increasing awareness that the transition to renewables has to be just. Unless they consider employment, affordability, and democratic involvement, green initiatives will once again reenact the fossil-fuel era of extraction. Energy justice, then, is also the need to incorporate by procedure (e.g., community consultation on renewable projects), distributional fairness (e.g., ensuring access to solar infrastructure), and recognizing systems of local knowledge as valid forms of expertise. These empirical observations are meant to bring out one thing again: that injustice in the environment is multidimensional. It requires more than direct technical evaluations of emissions or exposure. It also necessitates long-term participation in the histories, identities, and governance forms through which risks and benefits of ecology are apportioned.

Normative Tensions

There are underlying philosophical tensions that manifest in the presence of empirical patterns and policy debating such as between ecocentrism and anthropocentrism. According to ecocentric strategies, such as Deep Ecology (Naess, 2009) and biospheric egalitarianism, introduced by Arne Naess, it is claimed that it is the nonhuman life that has its intrinsic value and that justice must apply also to animals and ecosystems and even to the biosphere itself. In anthropocentric models, on the other hand, there is a high appraisal of nature as a means of human flourishing, where environmental conservation can be defined as an instrument toward human goals. Although ecocentrism provides this radical extension of the moral community, skeptics caution that it inadvertently disenfranchises human interests, specifically those of the most vulnerable of the vulnerable. In such a case, a heavy-handed policy of biodiversity conservation might rationalize the forcible removal of the Indigenous population off their ancestral territories, e.g., to increase biodiversity levels, thus continuing some traditions of colonial dispossession in the interest of environmental propriety. In this case, justice has to relate the inherent interests of nonhuman beings to the rights and welfare of the marginalized human communities. Intergenerational justice adds another layer of complexity. Assuming that justice involves treating the moral equality of human beings, then it should also consider those yet to be born. The approaches developed by philosophers as Parfit (1984) and Barry (1999) to argue that present generations have moral responsibilities to future ones within a nonidentity approach can be represented as the view that there exists a prudential rule, the so-called just savings principle advocated in the works mentioned by Rawls. There is, however, an underlying assumption in such frameworks that the future generation will have the same set of moral priorities that we do. They can indeed entail environmental destruction, economic development, and technological innovation in procedures which we cannot determine, as yet.

These intergenerational obligations are supposed to be a kind of channeled through sustainability metrics, which are also coming under fire. Although other measures such as Bhutan Gross National Happiness index or Ecological Footprint Analysis attempt to widen the range of the evaluation, Cartwright and Hardie (2012) make such warning that by aiming at quantification, epistemic closure can be regarded with the level of measuring something being more important than what is morally valuable. The danger is that such rich, qualitative ways of understanding ecological loss as the cultural significance of the disappearing scene lie erased in the script, since they cannot be incorporated according to uniform criteria. Environmental justice has to be philosophically sound must thus be wary of being seduced by numerical sufficiency. It must be epistemically pluralistic, historically accountable, and normatively reflexive. This implies considering the possibilities of knowing in more than one way, recognition of the historical exploitation tendencies, and readiness to redefine the ethical priorities when faced with new challenges.

The only thing is that justice in the environmental field is not a signing of climate agreements or working through sustainability checklists. It has to be rooted in ecological solidarity, seeing the connections between all forms of life, the inequities of power and accountability in international environmental politics, and the necessity of reparatory and preventive work. The environments need to be advocated justice by recasting political institutions, stretching the ethical circle and redesigning economic paradigms in such a way that they support rather than destroy the life-support systems of the planet. The present injustice to the Earth is, inevitably, injustice among the most vulnerable and also among those whose life has not even started.

Cross-Sectoral Intersectionality: Compound Injustices and Policy Synergies

The issues of health, education, and the environment are quite regularly addressed in a siloed ways of policy-making, with the implication that none of them is dependent upon the other. However, a closer look at empirical evidence as well as normative theory shows that they are profoundly intertwined. Intersectional disadvantage thus requires a cross-sectoral theory of justice: a situation where a range of social determinants of marginality mutually support each other and intensify that support, impossible to reduce to a linear cause and effect. The vulnerability is not merely additive; rather it is a co-constitutive as demonstrated in the foundation work of Kimberlene Crenshaw (1989) on intersectionality. The environmental precarity, educational marginalization, and health risks intertwine with the life of a girl living in a flood-prone informal settlement. They do not comprise various unique and individual misfortunes that unfortunately are experienced in tandem; they are structurally bound up with one another and each contributes to the harshness of the other. The solution to this according to the work is that in these situations, the isolation of the problem of health and the problem of environment or the problem of education does not only distort the actual reality of the afflicted individual but also has the potential of achieving ineffectual or even the reverse of sound policy results.

The integrative model of justice, which combines distribution, recognition, and representation components provided by Nancy Fraser (2009) can be viewed as a potent framework in terms of comprehending the fact that these areas support injustice when interrelated. The issue of distribution relates to material resources (clean water, school facility, and health care facilities). Recognition entails validation of marginalized groups aiding to their dignity and identity inclusive of the cultural, linguistic, as well as ecological knowledge. Representation means that those being acted upon are active participants in the decision-making concerning policies affecting their lives.

The Global South empirical research demonstrates the co-constitution of sector disparities. Low education achievement is highly related to low health indicators particularly in climate-stressed areas where there is dearth of clean water and sanitation. In these backgrounds, health risks are reinforced through educational marginalization that restricts health literacy and access to decent work and weakens resilience to environmental shocks. In a similar way, failing to educate students about environmental awareness through the curricula can be discussed as contributing to the phenomenon of ecological vulnerability and epistemic marginalization when societies struggle to educate youth on eco-systemic resilience.

Gendered and Racialized Experiences Across Sectors

It is impossible to pursue justice in any field without considering gender and race as the most basic dimensions of structural differentiation. In health, women and gender minorities frequently have disproportionately high levels of reproductive responsibilities, increased rates of gender-based violence, and de-facto underrepresentation in medical studies (Nussbaum, 2012; Crenshaw, 1991). These drawbacks are exacerbated where issues of environmental degeneration exist such as women having to go longer distances to obtain water or fuel as a result of environmental erosion thus subjecting them to the risks of physical injury or being held back by time poverty that restricts their educational and economic access. Educational inequities are also profoundly gendered and racialized. Girls in most regions of the world are handicapped in access to education due to the prevailing norms of patriarchy, privileging the education of boys and safety when going to school. The queer and trans young people face curricular erasures, antagonizing peer groups, and institutionalized discrimination that interferes with school success as well as mental health.

The racialized exposure patterns also shape the environmental sector. A study conducted by Robert Bullard (1993) on environmental racism details how polluting businesses are successfully located in communities of color. These environmental impacts combine with political weaknesses to oppose such siting decisions or to be able to require remediation. Specifically, indigenous women have a complicated role since they can be assigned as ecological custodians who preserve biodiversity and safeguard land and at the same time are exposed as some of the most vulnerable to environmental degradation. It is not only the livelihood of people who are threatened by land loss, exodus as the result of climate change, and loss of biodiversity, but also the cultural heritage and sovereignty.

The interdependency of injustice among these areas of oppression implies that, injustice is not only sectoral injustice and injustice is relational and historic. In philosophical terms, it requires going beyond formal equality, by which everyone is treated the same, and toward substantive and intersectionally conscious justice that meets the lived experience of cumulative disadvantage. This necessitates the need to base justice on abilities and cultural recognition so that the interventions ought to increase freedoms that are real and should respect various forms of knowledge and identity.

Integrated Justice Frameworks: From Siloed Policies to Multidimensional Interventions

Departmental compartmentalization has become synonymous with public policy, and the separation between the ministries of health, education, and environment has created a parallel world that in many instances lacks real coordination. This is not only ineffective, but also unjust since it does not pay attention to how deficits in one area limit advances in others. A holistic justice system acknowledges and seeks to overcome the compounding of sectoral disadvantages. The description of development as an enlargement of freedoms (Amartya Sen, 1999) provides a promising normative point of departure: lack of freedom in one area, say, education, denies other freedoms, such as the capacity to stay healthy, engage in sustainable livelihoods, or to engage in political affairs. This position is complemented by that of Martha Nussbaum (2013), who in the capabilities approach provides an orderly list of human capabilities, including bodily health, affiliation, and control over the environment as examples, which can be utilized in any domain to evaluate and enhance justice. This integration exemplifies the relational turn in theories of justice, which argues (Young, 2022) that people are not viewed as values-maximizing, independent individuals but as differently embedded subjects whose chances and welfare are tied to various movements of institutional arrangements. This school of thought changes the view of justice where the goal of justice revolves around the restoration of the individual gaps to a revolutionary focus on the institutions that create and perpetuate inequality.

Synergistic Policy Action: Contingent Transfers, Eco-Pedagogy, and Green Social Contracts

There are a couple of policy innovations that already reflect intersectional thinking although it is not necessarily articulated in those terms. Conditional cash transfer schemes (Brazillian Bolsa famila and Mexican progresa/Oportunidades) bridge the gap between education and health by paying cash to those families who guarantee the presence of their children at school and regular medical check-ups. These programs are open to criticism concerning their possible paternalism and surveillance, which encourages these programs to demonstrate that cross-sector alignment of incentives can deliver compounded benefits, disrupting cycles of deprivation in ways that atomized single-sector interventions cannot. Eco-pedagogy offers another model of cross-sectoral integration. Informed by the critical pedagogy of Paulo Freire (1970) and other scholars (e.g., Richard Kahn, 2010) and specifically informed by contemporary environmental problems, eco-pedagogy is a strategy or approach to education that ensures that the issues of environmental awareness such as the cultivation of ecological citizenship and values like sustainability, justice, and solidarity of the planet are embedded in educational curricula. This strategy is targeting not only environmental literacy but also to think critically around the social and political system that creates ecological damage and hence a connection between education, environment, and civic engagement.

The idea of the green social contract with references made by recent policy reports like the 2021 United Nations Development Programme report redefines the relationship between citizens and the state regarding the climate crisis. This framework asserts that social rights to health, education, and work should be reconciled with ecological sustainability so that current generation is not compromising the future at the expense of the future generations. Philosophically, this can be described as an extension of Rawlsian ideas of just collaboration in terms of covering not only the relations between generations but also the moral regard to nonhuman life.

These instances are a demonstration that justice is most efficient when taken as a systemic ethic as opposed to an administrative end. It is not merely to maximize efficiency or performance in the sector, but to change the moral structure of public policy so that equity, participation, and ecological responsibility will be routinely and systematically put in place. Finally, philosophically persuasive and empirically responsive justice should address intersecting systems of disadvantage that permeate health, education, and environment. In this context, Intersectionality is not just a descriptive phenomenon, but it is an epistemological approach, a normative perspective, and a framework of policy design. It is through the cultivation of intersectional moral imagination that we will be able to transcend piecemeal forms of interventionism and the establishment of an all-inclusive theory of structural fairness, a theory that embraces the dignity of not only human flourishing but also of ecological flourishing.

Institutional Ethics and Democratic Accountability

The fundamental problem of any utilitarian-cognitive version of justice is whether or not institutions are functional programs of justice or simply mechanisms of reproduction of inequality. This issue, stated by Iris Marion Young (2022) and Nancy Fraser (2009), describes the equivocal character of institutions as means and possible impediments to justice. Institutions, more broadly, we may talk of legal systems, bureaucracies, educational frameworks, health infrastructures, and environmental agencies, do not merely administer norms but form them. They define the parameters of the recognitions, resource allocation, and the ability to be included. Institutions turn out to be sources of misrecognition and distributive injustice when they incorporate structural biases like racism, classism, patriarchy, or colonial legacies into their design (Fraser, 2009).

Institutional ethics hence goes beyond process justice to dive into some of the underlying ontological premises and ecological political geographies that institutions replicate. In defining basic institutions, most prominently the main object of justice (Rawls, 1999), John Rawls reminds of their fundamental contribution to the life prospects. However, his view of the well-governed society presented in idealized models tends to overlook the inertia, vested interests, and political capture that may make institutions morally opaque or even actively exclusionary. This is because real-world justice demands that normative examination be constantly applied to institutions of justice-asking not just about their compliance with formal standards, but whether they are engaged in dismantling or reinforcing systemic injustice.

Democratic Participation in Policy Design: Whose Voices Count?

The institutional legitimacy of deliberation raises one of the major issues of institutional ethics: who speaks, and who listens? This is not because democratic participation in policy design is merely a procedural ideal but rather a substantive norm of justice, based on the principle of equal moral worth and epistemic reciprocity. In line with Habermas (1996) and Sen (2009), the democratic legitimacy is revealed when norms are justified publicly through deliberation based on reasons that free and equal citizens obtain. However, across several domains of policy formulation, especially in health, education, and environmental policies, spaces of decision-making are technocratic in their representation, or tokenistic in nature rendering those who stand most impacted by the consequences as others. The women of rural economies, the Indigenous peoples in climatically vulnerable regions, and the poor urban residents often have minimal access to influencing the institutions to which their livelihoods are subjected. This is an epistemic injustice, as Sandra Harding (2008) and Boaventura de Sousa Santos (2014) note: the exclusion of some knowledges not because they are untrue or irrelevant but because they have been dismissed as less authoritative under the existing hierarchies of power. Substantive participation involves coming out of consultation to co-creation, where communities contribute in problem definition, solution generation, and evaluation criteria. Without such a degree of participation, participatory rhetoric will merely be hiding the persistence of an unequal balance of power. The ability of the institutions to allow communities to set the agenda and by establishing the standards is the only way that the institutions can claim the ethical legitimacy of acting as agents of justice and not as actors of injustice.

Indicators and Public Reasoning in Sectoral Governance

Accountability often comes through indicators, that is, quantitative and qualitative measures aimed at monitoring performance, equity, and inclusion in institutions. However, by pointing to the possible indicators, it is not advisable to view these indicators as ends in themselves, as a capability-based theory of justice postulates (Sen, 2009). They are a means to an end, not alternatives to it, to help with reasoning in the public. Indicators should be contestable, revised, and interpretable in context. As in the case of the education index, which only takes into consideration enrolment rates that masks the gendered patterns of dropout, or the health equity measure, which may not reflect the burden of unpaid care giving or inequality in accessing reproductive health resources. The success of any indicator is gauged by its moral clarity, inclusiveness, and sensitivity to different values. This reframing challenges the technocratic ideal of neutral measurement. The normative assumptions in models and metrics, as Cartwright and Hardie (2012) remark, have to be made explicit to facilitate the ethical assessment of the framework. In sectoral governance, performance is assessed and managed through indicators directing resource distribution, guaranteeing conformity, and measuring performance. However, in the absence of deliberative legitimacy they can become the tools of administrative abstraction: The pursuit of outputs rather than the confrontation of the reality of injustice that they purport to quantify. Ethically strong indicators arise when their construction is participatory, their categories anticipate plural epistemologies, and the application of the indicators elicits corrective action following the recognition of the inequities found out. In this regard, indicators do not just act as instruments of governance, but may become triggers to democratic accountability.

Transparency, Accountability, and Moral Legitimacy

Transparency and accountability are commonly praised as major essentials of good government, but the normative implications of these concepts is less commonly considered. Transparency does not simply mean the disclosure of information; rather it makes power visible and subject to accountability. Accountability entails more than just delivery on performance standards, it is the requirement to explain the institutional conduct in acceptable terms to those who are influenced by it. According to Bovens (2007), it is possible to tell the difference between accountability as control, accountability as dialogue, and accountability as learning. The normative aspect of accountability is brought into the picture when it is instilled as of democratic norms so that it is not just outfitted that accountability institutions are merely answerable on consequences but also open to criticism and capable of reformation. For instance, a school board is responsible not only of test scores but also for issues like whether their policies reflect community values, of whether their decision-making addresses past injustices, and whether they uphold pedagogical integrity.

Moral legitimacy cannot be conferred by procedural checklists alone. This relies on the perceptions of people whether institutions are just, inclusive, and respectful of various moral claims. The theory of recognitional ethics by Axel Honneth (1995) associates legitimacy with the continual postwar recognition of individuals and communities as complete moral subjects. This requires the institutions to be in constant processes of justification, critique, and modification to retain the faithfulness of people. Institutional legitimacy is thus relational and dynamic. It is maintained by the epistemic openness, participatory design, and ethical responsiveness. The fact that an institution is morally inert is wrong; it is a place where normal work, identity formation, and resource allocation happens. They can also become agents of justice when they are deliberatively open, when they acknowledge plural epistemologies, and when they are morally accountable. By obscuring, marginalizing, or technocratizing decision-making, they run the risk of reproducing injustice in the name of governance.

The design and participation and measurement and legitimacy as moral imperatives must be built into a philosophical reconstruction of institutions as something more than an administrative consideration at the end of the process. This reconstruction needs a shift wherein the entrenched notions of compliance models are changed in favor of adaptive frameworks that are reflexive to criticism and sensitive to the changing ideas of justice. Institutions, together with their democratic accountability or their ethical self-examination, are the only means that can turn them into instruments of human dignity and ecological sustainability, infusing democratic accountability and normative self-scrutiny into their very core.

Concluding Summary

In bringing this adventure into the sectoral indwelling of justice through health, education, and environmental policy, we must be against the vice of reifying justice to the issue of fair distribution alone. It is impossible to deny the importance of distributive fairness, of who gets what, and in what quantity. However, a framework that concentrates on distribution would be an ethically inferior one in case it cannot question the structural mechanisms, which produce inequality over and over again.

Structural injustice is not, as Iris Marion Young (1990) explained, simply an aggregation of institutionally unjust actions (acts of maldistribution), but instead it consists of a systemic set of arrangements of institutionalized norms, economic relationships, cultural devaluations, and political exclusions. The only solution would be to address injustice by going beyond the renunciation of goods under the face of the old norms and confronting the methods by which the old norms themselves reproduce asymmetry. Health care is unjust when unequal access occurs, but also when the social determinants of health such as housing, environmental safety, and nutrition are created by logics of exclusion. It is interesting to mention that injustice in education occurs not onlywhen resources are distributed unequally, but also when curriculum reinforces colonial knowledge systems or patriarchal epistemologies that depreciate other forms of knowledge.

The sectoral justice, thus, should shift in its aims fixed on the amelioration of outcomes to the aims on building a brand new social scaffolding in order to accomplish these outcomes. Justice in this philosophical mode is not a rectifying piecework but a dislocating and constructive program, the recasting of institutions, collective imaginaries, and social relations. The technocratization of justice is one of the frequent risks of modern policy discourse: the idea that any social issue can be solved by optimal indicators, models, and algorithms. This trend can actually be seen in the growth of justice metrics, which, although invaluable in terms of transparency and accountability, can unwittingly push the moral compass of justice out of sight.

Today, as Amartya Sen (2009) reminds us, measurement must be subject to informed and open debate, as well as to be based on the pluralism of moral visions of those involved. The quantitative clarity becomes fetishized in danger of forgetting about qualitative aspects of human life: metrics can tell how many kids go to school but cannot describe what they are being taught or the ways in which their dignity is being constructed; they can quantify carbon footprints but not ecological grief or cultural dispossession. The issue, in other words, is not the despondent acceptance of policy tools, but the re-enchantment of policy tools with moral imagination, as Martha Nussbaum (2013) defines it: the ability to view other people as ends-in-themselves, having histories and struggles, their own as well as ours. The moral imagination guards against the suffocation of calculation and provides room to make decisions through policies that are ethically dense, culturally conscious, and politically reflective. It makes sure that numbers are never used as justice itself.

In this sense, policy is not simply the application of previously established norms but rather a field of normative inquiry and judgment, where justice should be understood, debated, and achieved by reference to the requirements or challenges of rapidly changing realities. This necessitates epistemic humility: the recognition that no single paradigm or measure can adequately represent all aspects of human well-being and ecological health. And it needs philosophical boldness: the ability to reconsider established categories, to give hearing to the voices at the margins, and to think differently about possible futures. This chapter has shown that justice as it is applied to areas of sectoral activity must operate between normative aspiration and empirical limit. It should not dwell only on what is good but also on what is practicable, quantifiable, and politically challengeable. This tension raises the more fundamental philosophical question called out by this work in the next chapter to investigate what kinds of measures constitute and are the measure of justice and why it matters.

Justice metrics are double-edged tools. They have the ability to shed light on socially hidden injustices and trigger remedial public policy measures and democratizing the production of knowledge. They can however also deepen normative reductionism, insist on the superiority of abstraction to concrete experience, and push down goods which cannot be measured. The policy models are never neutral in reference to morality, as they delineate certain presumptions regarding human value, social causation, and action legitimacy. Questions of whether justice can or should become an indicator or whether it needs to remain a meta-norm that is not fully quantifiable will then be asked in the next chapter. It will look at the philosophical preconditions to such a view: how might indicators be formulated that will understand moral texture without formalizing justice? How can the empirical instruments be normatively embedded without being subordinate to the needs of governance?

The chapter reinstates the importance of the philosophical involvement in the empirical methodologies in taking that step by moving away with sectoral analysis toward an exploration of the meta-theoretical reflection. This is not returning to practice but rather an in-depth engagement in the ideas of ethical concepts on which governance exists. It acknowledges that the way we quantify justice determines the way we seek justice, that measurement not only misleads our statistics but our ethics as well. The moral horizon in this case transcends onto enhanced metrics or more effective policies. It hopes in transformative justice, a normative mood that aims at redefining the infrastructures of feasibility in human and environmental thriving. This can only be achieved through the ethical rebuilding of the institutions of the polity, through the crafting of indicators as objects of democratic critique as opposed to administrative measures, and by injecting policy with liberatory perspective.

In accordance with the argument provided by Fraser (2009) and de Sousa Santos (2014), the notion of justice as a concept requires our epistemic plurality and political imagination: the ability both to criticize the system hegemonic knowledge and to imagine new models of solidarity, inclusion, and sustainability. The work of justice in a world cleaved apart by widening inequality, climate catastrophe, and continuing epistemic subjection is, then, neither just to maintain that present nor to preserve that status quo. Justice must do more than live in the present, mere management of it. Justice must work to ensure rather a more dignified, participatory, and ecologically cancerous future. In this sense, justice is not merely a policy outcome. It is a continuing moral practice, a form of collective reasoning, and a philosophical provocation, one that is never quite resolved, never so done, always requiring renewal, and yet desperately needed in our time.

References

Anderson, E. (2007). Fair opportunity in education: A democratic equality perspective. *Ethics, 117*(4), 595–622.

Anderson, E. (2013). *The imperative of integration*. Princeton University Press.

Barry, B. (1999). Sustainability and intergenerational justice. In A. Dobson (Ed.), *Fairness and futurity: Essays on environmental sustainability and social justice*. Oxford University Press.

bell hooks. (1994). *Teaching to transgress: Education as the practice of freedom*. Routledge.

Bovens, M. (2007). Analysing and assessing accountability: A conceptual framework. *European Law Journal, 13*(4), 447–468.

Bullard, R. D. (1993). Confronting environmental racism: Voices from the grassroots. South End Press.

Caney, S. (2010). Climate change and the duties of the advantaged. *Critical Review of International Social and Political Philosophy, 13*(1), 203–228.

Crenshaw, K. (1989). Demarginalizing the intersection of race and sex. *University of Chicago Legal Forum*, 139–167.

Daniels, N. (2008). *Just health: Meeting health needs fairly*. Cambridge University Press.

Deshpande, S. (2014). *The problem of caste*. Orient Blackswan.

Fraser, N. (2009). *Scales of justice: Reimagining political space in a globalizing world*. Columbia University Press.

Freire, P. (1970). *Pedagogy of the oppressed*. Herder and Herder.

Gutmann, A. (1999). *Democratic education* (Review ed.). Princeton University Press.

Harding, S. (2008). *Sciences from below: Feminisms, postcolonialities, and modernities*. Duke University Press.

Honneth, A. (1995). *The struggle for recognition: The moral grammar of social conflicts*. MIT Press.

Kahn, R. (2010). *Critical pedagogy, ecoliteracy, and planetary crisis*. Peter Lang.

Naess, A. (2009). *Ecology, community and lifestyle: Outline of an ecosophy*. Cambridge University Press.

Nixon, R. (2013). *Slow violence and the environmentalism of the poor*. Harvard University Press.

Nussbaum, M. C. (2012). *Women and human development: The capabilities approach*. Cambridge University Press.

Nussbaum, M. C. (2013). *Creating capabilities: The human development approach*. Harvard University Press.

Michalos, A. C., & Hatch, P. M. (2020). Good societies, financial inequality and secrecy, and a good life: From Aristotle to Piketty. *Applied Research in Quality of Life, 15*(3), 1005–1054. https://doi.org/10.1007/s11482-019-09717-0

Parfit, D. (1984). *Reasons and persons*. Oxford University Press.

Rawls, J. (1971). *A theory of justice*. Harvard University Press.

Rawls, J. (1999). *A theory of justice* (Review ed.). Harvard University Press.

Santos, B. d. S. (2014). *Epistemologies of the south: Justice against epistemicide*. Routledge.

Schlosberg, D. (2007). Defining environmental justice: Theories, movements, and nature. Oxford University Press.

Sen, A. (1999). *Development as freedom*. Oxford University Press.

Sen, A. (2002). Health: Perception versus observation. *BMJ, 324*(7342), 860–861.

Sen, A. (2009). *The idea of justice*. Harvard University Press.

Skutnabb-Kangas, T. (2013). *Linguistic genocide in education—or worldwide diversity and human rights?* Lawrence Erlbaum.

Tuck, E., & Yang, K. W. (2012). Decolonization is not a metaphor. *Decolonization: Indigeneity, Education & Society, 1*(1).

Young, I. M. (2022). *Justice and the politics of difference*. Princeton University Press.

Chapter 7
Philosophical Reflections on Justice Metrics

Introduction: Why Metrics Need Philosophy

It is in the context of this regime of quantification-as-governance that justice itself is being converted into a measurable dimension, captured in rates of access, equity gaps, inclusion measures, and participatory ratios. This change does not occur at the methodological levels; it also symbolizes a more fundamental moral change. Justice, long upheld in the contemplation of philosophers and reasoning of ethics, is currently considered as a technocratic item of provision. The opening of this chapter is easy to remember but is a heavy thought: Is justice measurable without being diminished? It enquires as to whether the operationalization of justice through indicators, i.e., what one can call justice metrics, empowers justice or impoverishes it in a subtle manner. Although indicators are able to add epistemic clarity, accountability, and comparability, they do face the possibility of moral simplification, conceptual distortion, and loss of values that do not lend themselves easily to quantification. Whether to use metrics is no longer even a question, but how to construct and interpret them in a manner that is ethically responsible and epistemologically self-critical is its main consideration.

Indicators and the Technocratic Turn in Justice Discourse

The emergence of justice measures has to be nested in the more general process of datafication of government. The Sustainable Development Goals by the UN, inequality dashboards at the country level, and the use of indicators as tools of diagnosis, benchmarking, and policy correction are all deployed. The rationale behind the attraction of quantification is, as Theodore M. Porter (2020) puts it, its ability to promise the objectivity of mechanics; that is, that quantifications produce

S. K. Maurya, *Exploring Justice as a Social Indicator of Life*, Social Indicators Research Series 92, https://doi.org/10.1007/978-3-032-10812-8_7

value-free, reproducible, and auditable data. What was said is given moral high stakes when applied to justice. Indicators seem to anchor such idealized normative concepts in empirical verifiability, offering a sense of assurance that justice and equity can be measured in the same way as budget deficits or literacy levels. Yet, this impression of neutrality is misleading. Because of thick ethical concepts involved that are both descriptive and evaluative, the policy measures always involve thick ethical terms, like, fair, inclusive, or equitable, as Nancy Cartwright and Jeremy Hardie (2015) support. The creation of an indicator of justice is never neutral technical exercise; it bears a code on what would be considered just, which voices are to be taken into account, and what ultimate consequences will be prioritized. In this sense, justice measures are not impartial ways to look at the world. They are enmeshed in political and moral views of the world, and inform the way problems are defined, the set of solutions that are available, and what success consists of.

The Philosophical Task: Interrogating Metrics as Moral Constructs

These questions span multiple philosophical traditions. The arguments are intertwined with those over-conceptual analysis, value commensurability, and indexical meaning, which are debated in the analytic philosophy (Anderson, 1993; Sen, 2009). They are associated, in the thinking of the continent, with critiques of technocracy and instrumental reason, and of the colonization of the lifeworld (Habermas, 1987; Foucault, 1978). Through either of the accounts, the warning is similar: Unless one pays special attention to the metrics applications in justice talk, the stated threat involves the transformation of ethical discussion into a mathematical policy. The solution however is not to lapse into anti-metric romanticism. Indicators are part and parcel of the modern mode of governance such that they cannot be left behind. The work of philosophy is to rebuild them: to contextualize them with notions of moral rivalry, democratic argument, and epistemic diversity. Measurements are not to be tested merely on statistical grounds of validity, but also on grounds of normative-sense, i.e., the ways they are being open to reinterpretation, or empowering those who they are being measured, rather than masking their realities.

Justice Metrics as Ethically Charged Instruments

Justice measures are morally loaded tools, the validity of which is determined by more than technical precision. They should be appraised in terms of their morality transparency, democratic accountability, and inclusiveness. What standardized indicators omit, rather than disclose, is the critical ethical question: What types of knowledge, experience, and value are left out in the cold? Who sets the parameters in which measurements are made and to whose interest are these parameters determined? The capability approach by Amartya Sen, 2009 provides a form of resourceful counterbalance to reductionism. According to Sen, plurality of informational space is critical in assessing justice and will not support the use of any particular measure, income, utility, or access, as a measure of well-being. To him, even the indicator developing process must be a place of justice, where different people, particularly marginal groups, are included in the establishment of evaluation standards. Such a deliberative focus does not treat indicators as pronouncement but as starting points of continued public deliberation, which should at all times be contentious, subject to revision and new knowledge. Through which the justice measures may be renegotiated within the logic of dynamic moral forms as opposed to technical outputs. Rather, they are turned into channels of democracy of communication rather than bureaucratic seals.

Philosophy's Role in the Era of Measurement

Justice metrics do not only count because they are a new form of governmental instrumentality, but because it is a new form of doing moral mediation. They are seated at the crossroad between normative ideals and empiricism, between the transformation of normative ideals into operational categories, and between the ideals of democracy and the limitations on knowledge imposed by the quantification. The philosophical problem is how to make a middle way between these two dangers: the impoverishment of justice to what can be measured, and the devaluation of measuring that there is anything corrupting about measurement. One cannot measure justice without misshaping it but one cannot forego measurement without running the risk of neglecting justice altogether. The challenge then is to devise a philosophy of ethical or normative measurement, one that acknowledges the irreducibility of justice on the one hand, and creates instruments that are morally opaque, epistemically inclusive, and politically answerable. This can only be achieved by struggling against the lures of mechanical objectivity by paying due respect to the fact that all metrics were moral assertions in disguise. It involves as well the development of moral imagination: vision of what is not yet registered in existing measures, foresight of new forms of injustice, and vision of other ways of knowing and valuing.

This chapter sets out to advance such a framework. It will shift between the normative and the empirical, abstraction and detail, in the effort to address the question of how justice can be made operational without being trivialized. The discourse will cover the duality of indicators as both an empirical and normative argument and the ways in which they have potential to uncover the superseded inequities on the one hand and the tendency to conceal the moral complexity of a problem. The chapter engages in the questioning of justice of metrics and the metrics of justice with the purposes of dislodging measurement as a technocratic activity to highlighting it as an ethically reflexive one. Thereby, it encourages policy-makers, scholars, and citizens to view metrics less as the final point of moral argument and more as its starting point a common tongue with which we can argue, bargain, and otherwise hone our mutual visions of what it means to be an ethical society.

The Ontology of Justice and the Problem of Quantification

The quantification of justice presents a profound ontological paradox. On the one hand, justice is one of the greatest values in moral philosophy and political theory, which is now operationalized in the whenever possible quantitative terms: in equity scores, fairness indices, accessibility rates, and rights-based measures. Conversely, justice as a normative ideal, as a second-order value, as a historically changing moral orientation has its own resistance to be easily objectified. To attempt to measure justice is thus to commit the error of carrying a category mistake: of reducing to a set of measurable surrogates morally complex, qualitatively rich concepts.

Is Justice a Measurable Entity or a Regulative Ideal?

According to Kant, justice is a regulative ideal; a horizon of concepts that we can never reach, but can only work on as such. Kant's moral law, grounded in the categorical imperative, is not empirically derived but a priori, shaping the moral orientation of rational agents (Kant, 1785/1996). Such a view of justice does not present it as an empirical datum that can be measured with a survey instrument; rather, justice is a guiding normativity, a standard that can never be reached, it frames criticism, transformation, and hope. In the same way, John Rawls in *A Theory of Justice* has considered justice in the form of fairness to be a principle guiding the constitution of institutions and not the characteristic feature of isolated outcomes that may be quantified in terms of numbers. His thought experiments, the original position and the veil of ignorance, place justice in the realm of evaluative frameworks rather than as a variable to be inserted into a social science regression line (Rawls, 1971).

To some degree, the temptation to treat justice as something that can be measured is the result of positivist and utilitarian traditions, which tend to conflate normative ideals with empirical indicators. This shift however calls into question basic ontological issues: What is the nature of justice? Is it a property, a relation, a disposition? Can it be instantiated, detected, or indexed? Anywhere in the world is it mediated by interpretation, discourse and historical context? These questions are not all abstract since each will regulate whether we are measuring justice, or only the semblance of it.

The Ontological Gap Between Moral Value and Empirical Proxy

Ontological gap is central to this dilemma, the structural disjuncture between the moral ontology of justice, on the one hand, and the epistemic practices of measurement, on the other. Indicators can help bring into focus some institutional or experiential aspects of wrongs, unequal sentencing rates or disparities in educational opportunities, but they do so by stripping the context, meaning, and difficulty that give particular injustices their full ethical significance. For instance, consider the case of healthcare access. A health equity index, which monitored differences in service usage by the demographic group. While such information as important as it cannot capture the lived experiences of dignity, vulnerability, or recognition during a clinical interaction. Nor does it readily reflect the impacts of historical marginalization, intergenerational trauma, or symbolic exclusion. As Nancy Fraser (2009) emphasizes, justice is not reducible to distribution alone; it also entails recognition and political representation, dimensions that often escape numeric abstraction.

Epistemic pluralism, in turn, contributes to distinct cultures, groups, and philosophies have varying ideas about how to think about justice itself in redistributive, reparative, reciprocal or responsible terms. A single global indicator cannot accommodate these incommensurable visions without engaging in ontological flattening or, worse, normative imperialism (Santos, 2014).

Justice is not a concrete object like clean water or good housing, not a first-order commodity but a second-order appraisal notion. Justice informs us on the distribution, decision-making, and treatment of persons. Measuring justice is, thus, the effort to gauge the circumstances in which moral relations are properly organized. It brings the risk of a category mistake, a concept from Gilbert Ryle (1949) referring to the attribution of a property to something that cannot logically have it. By establishing a justice index, when policy-makers combine indicators (income equality, representation in decision-making, and public trust), the result may create an implicit notion of justice as a totality of these aspects, when it is actually a criterion, upon which such aspects are measured. This collapses evaluative constructions with such empirical sums and dangers reification: making a relationship ideal seem like a separate thing. Elizabeth Anderson (1993) cautions that justice involves "thick ethical concepts" that blend factual and evaluative content. The subversion of such concepts into separate and measurable traits does not attain an effective level without sacrificing its normative richness. It is not possible for the subversion of such concepts into distinct and quantifiable qualities to reach an effective level without loss of its normative richness. In that regard, metrics could never be complete manifestations, at best divulgers of justice as a symptom, but not substance.

The Philosophical Stakes of Measuring Normative Concepts

Modern instrumental rationality of contemporary governance contributes to the evolution of the modern attempt to measure justice. According to the logic of administration, the things that are not measurable are easily unable to be taken, as actionable. In this context, justice turns out to be a technical variable the purpose of which is to be optimized, ranked, and benchmarked.

Philosophically, this shift is consequential:

- Depoliticization: As Jacques Rancière (2004) argues, politics begins where disagreement over the meaning of justice emerges. The problem with metrics is that they risk silencing such disagreements with the impression of justice as fixed and not a candidate to dispute.
- Moral Disengagement: Moral arguments are replaced by mathematical standards, as in the case where enhancing a Gini coefficient is considered as a form of ethical performance where a Gini coefficient of less than 0.3 will be taken to contain the society in question as fair.
- Epistemic Injustice: Drawing from Miranda Fricker's (2007) concept of hermeneutical injustice, metrics based on dominant frameworks may fail to recognize or express marginalized communities' own understandings of justice, thereby erasing alternative epistemologies.
- Path Dependency: Indicators shape institutional priorities. Measuring justice one way is to favor one form of injustice against another, although usually unwittingly, with long-term effects.

So the issue is not just that justice is a hard thing to quantify, that quantification is itself a value-laden, morally significant, and philosophically contentious activity.

Toward an Ontologically Responsible Philosophy of Measurement

It is equally impractical and undesirable to eschew indicators completely as they bear too much promise of revealing deep-seated unfairness and tracing institutional responsibility. It is difficult to develop an ontologically responsible approach to measurement, which does not lose the qualitative fullness of justice out of sight, which regards the limits and constructed form of quantification.

This requires:

- The incorporation of metrics in deliberative mechanisms whereby such definitions and implications are subject to collective and open challenge.
- Designing indicators more suggestive of plural conceptions of justice as opposed to imposing a singular normative frame.
- The reliance on measurements as contingent indicators, rather than authoritative pronouncements, partly about the state of justice.

The retention of both the imperative and boundaries of measurement allows such a framework to turn the measures of justice into a weapons of democracy, rather than the tools of reduction. Measurement would go on to work justice, not to substitute moral deliberation, but to support and enrich it.

Indicators as Epistemic Authority

The rising indiscrimination of indicators in the policy of justice has altered governance and, behind the scenes, shifted the concept of what constitutes valid knowledge of justice. The shift in the world of moral thought away (a) from philosophical logic and normative argumentation to (b) numerical measurement has transformed the landscape of moral reflection: ethical statements are supposed to be proven by statistical data, and political assertions are to be reduced to measurable signs. This shift is not merely methodological, it is epistemological. It privileges certain types of knowledge over others, who gets to count as having experiences that really count, what is considered real, whose realities are considered, and what kinds of interventions are considered rational or actionable.

As Theodore Porter (2020) has argued, quantification draws its authority from the ideal of "mechanical objectivity"-the belief that numbers can speak independently of bias, ideology, or interpretive interference. This power is given exponentially greater moral significance in the context of justice: pointers are to place the moral ideals on empirical certainty, such that they can be measured, compared, and audited. Yet, as Sally Engle Merry (2011) reminds us, this process is never neutral. The indicators take what is essentially complex and multidimensional in social realities and reduces this to simplified numerical forms. Such a translation is bound to result into decisions of what to measure, how to measure, and whose opinions to consider.

This epistemic authority is double-edged. On the one hand, indicators can democratize knowledge by making the invisible patterns of inequality visibly apparent, as well as legitimizing the experiences of marginalized groups, and keeping powerful institutions accountable. The potential to make invisible the forms of life and suffering that cannot be easily compartmentalized, their ability to remove any level of complexity or eliminate ambivalence all come to the other side of reductiveness. Within the bureaucratic environment, what cannot be measured frequently does not become actionable, and thus, in practice, not actual. Indicators are thus not descriptive, they are prescriptive; they construct a version of reality one that is readable and understandable by systems of governance but which may also be foreign to the lives experienced by individuals being measured.

Objectivity, Bias, and Epistemic Exclusion

Indicators are sold to us as being objective, however, their purported neutrality is more than ideal. As feminist epistemologists like Helen Longino (1990) and Sandra Harding (1992) have demonstrated, all knowledge production is situated, shaped by social position, institutional context, and power relations. The indicator building process comprises several decisions, laden with value: what variables to use, which outcomes to focus on, what populations to sample, and what thresholds to establish. Such decisions have tacit assumptions of relevancy, causality, and normativity in them. Take, for instance, an "access to justice" index. Is right of access framed in response to the availability of legal aid, the intelligibility of legal systems based on cultural experience, or the sense of substantive justice in the procedure whereby one is the subject of that procedure? Every operational decision constitutes a specific ethical and political perception of the meaning of justice and how it is to be encountered. The formal equality before the law can mean a lot to one person and substantive to the other, the functionality in operating within the legal institutions. These alternative emphases do not exist as isolated issues of technical diversity, but rather as issues, which themselves contain some contentious conceptions of justice as such.

Furthermore, the biases associated with the design of indicators may dynamically play out in politically coded but highly significant ways. The data sets often underrepresent marginalized populations because of underreporting, misclassification, or infrastructural disregard, resulting in what would be described as statistical erasure. One way models can harm or hinder justice is by ensuring efficiency or cost-effectiveness over equity, thereby enforcing technocratic principles at the cost of justice. The hermeneutics themselves tend to privilege mainstream cultural explanations of fairness leaving aside local epistemologies, which could reframe the issue and solution. This leads directly to the problem of epistemic injustice, as articulated by Miranda Fricker (2007). It is possible that when the justice metrics are designed in such a way that does not involve the voices of the people being measured, there is a risk of engaging in a hermeneutical wrong, that of failing to reflect the meanings, experiences, and moral models of those being measured. The epistemology of Sandra Harding reinforces this conclusion further: knowledge is not produced by a gaze into nowhere but is produced by the standpoints in particular social positions, and in-group standpoints stop the blind spots of a dominant way of seeing reality. In the perspective of the oppressed, distinct evils become experientially real, distinguishing standards of equity arise, and distinct standards of evidentiary weight are recognized. These perspectives have not been captured in the design of indicators because it is not just a technical lapse, but a moral harm. Boaventura de Sousa Santos (2014) calls this epistemicide: the erasure of nondominant ways of knowing under the guise of scientific neutrality. The translation of this to the context of justice metrics imply that the existing institutions will not only dictate the language of evaluation but also the fact of legitimacy, i.e. what might be good justice in the first place.

Toward Epistemic Democracy in Justice Metrics

In order to be valid indicators tool in the policy arena of justice, indicators will have to be reconceptualized, not as constituting arbiters of reality but as tentative, disputable artifacts residing in democratic discussion. In this situation, the solution created by Amartya Sen regarding the idea of responsive reasoning is very attractive. In The Idea of Justice (2009), Sen critiques "transcendental institutionalism," the search for perfect principles detached from lived realities, and instead calls for comparative evaluations grounded in plural informational spaces. According to it, justice is not established in an irreversible way by abstract theory but is always reinterpreted by inclusive discussion. In this light, indicators are to be considered as an ethico-epistemic formation, or rather a hybrid of empirical observation and the moral assessment. Their validity cannot be measured merely in respect of statistical reliability, predictive power, they also have to be judged in regard to epistemic justice, interpretive inclusivity, and ethical intelligibility. The measure of justice is, in other words, to be judged not only in terms of how well it is an approximation of the number but also the extent of its design process, the explicitness of its assumptions, and its susceptibility to revision.

This requires a set of reforms. First, the development of participatory indicator must be institutionalized, and those it will impact the most need to be given significant power. Second, reflexive methodologies should work to clarify the normative commitments implicit in measurement decisions, recognizing their cultural and political contingency. Third, indicators must be coupled with qualitative accounts stories of people, ethnographies, oral histories, and case studies that reflect aspects of justice that cannot be seen by numerical proxies. Fourth, the interpretation should be context-sensitive, and the attempt to overgeneralize and present usually context-limited information should be avoided. The reforms of such a kind change the epistemic role of indicators appointed by the technocratic authorities to democratic interlocutors. Measurements are not in themselves the goals of this model but triggers of further reasoning in the public. They enter into a discussion that is ongoing regarding what justice is, how it must be sought, and how its achievement is to be assessed. The above-mentioned changes demand both epistemic humility, the idea that one or another metric cannot reveal the entire moral landscape of justice, and the pluralistic values of ways of knowing.

In the end, the aim should not be to abandon indicators wholesomely, but rather to reconstitute their epistemological role. Justice measures are neither to concentrate power nor to delegate entrusted responsibilities to empirical duties. Rather, they ought to be avenues of communication between evidence and assessment that would allow the societies to face the quantifiable and the the unquantifiable aspects of justice. That, given the tools we employ to know justice would be to develop and apply epistemic democracy: to take care to make sure that our means of knowing justice are in turn developed fairly and justly.

The Normative Architecture of Measurement

It is a starting point observation in the philosophy of science and political theory that measurement is never a neutral act. It always entails value judgments as to what is to be attended to, what is improvement or decline, and what trade-offs can be accepted. These judgments are especially significant in a social indicators field where the metrics selected tend to influence what parts of human activity is made visible within institutions and which are not. As Amartya Sen (1980) pointed out in his early critique of both utilitarianism and income-based measures, to decide what to measure is already to commit to a conception of the good. The supposed technical neutrality of statistical indicators has the following undertones of deep normativeness.

This is an entanglement of values that is left unspoken by the modern day government. It brings about indicators as unemotional, as an objective instrument, the purpose of which is to act as a factual basis of a decision. However, the way they are built never lacks any ethical, political, and epistemological premises. The calculation of any index, score, or ranking presupposes a vision: either explicit or implicit, of how the human condition is to be constituted and what it means to flourish. This chapter claims that indicators in categories like justice, health, and development are not only empirical instruments but moral constructions, and they carry specific constructions of the world even in cases where they are explicitly presented as much needed technical tools.

The Ethical Fabric of Metrics: What Does and Does Not Get Counted

It is at the selection of variables that normative commitments are most instant. All ratios are predicated on a more fundamental choice: what in life seems significant enough to measure. The Human Development Index (HDI) is a well-known example. It tracks education, life expectancy, and per capita income as its three pillars, thereby reflecting a broadly liberal economic view of well-being (UNDP, 1990). The things it does not measure politically and morally matter just as much (or, never mind, more), such practices as political freedom, cultural identity, environmental integrity, but such are not displayed by its statistics. This omission is not incidental, but transparent of the priorities and philosophical commitments of the designers of the metric. The Multidimensional Poverty Index (MPI) is more expansive, measuring deprivations in health, education, and living standards. However, as Alkire and Foster (2011) admit, the selection of these specific dimensions was driven by both empirical evidence and stakeholder values, as well as political feasibility, which explicitly articulates the normative selectivity of the exercise.. By contrast, Bhutan's Gross National Happiness (GNH) framework incorporates dimensions like spiritual well-being, community vitality, and environmental harmony. This broadened scope reflects Buddhist metaphysical commitments and communitarian ethics. Whereas the GNH is more encompassing and colorful, it provokes dilemmas related to cultural specificity and translation of such indicators into other contexts of political or moral value.

Elizabeth Anderson's (1993) concept of "thick ethical concepts" is useful here. Thick terms such as well-being or justice are messy: they cannot be split into factual description and moral judgment, but instead it is all part and parcel. The selection of the variables results in a metric that not only describes the state of the world, but which also defines a view of how the good life should be like. The failure to count conveys the implicit message that what is being excluded is not so important—the thinly disguised moral choice under the guise of methodological necessity.

Cartwright and Hardie on "Thick" Concepts in Policy Models

Nancy Cartwright and Jeremy Hardie (2015), in Evidence-Based Policy, offer one of the clearest critiques of the illusion of neutrality in measurement. They claim that policy models are constructed based on thick ethical concepts whose evaluative content cannot be discarded without distorting the content of the concepts. Concepts such as the notions of justice, empowerment, or resilience do not represent value-free terms; they are a moral judgment carried in words. These thick concepts are often operationalized into numerical variables that oversimplify or distort their meaning in many instances. Consider the example of a justice index that forfeits the great effects of justice to three dimensions, access, representation, and transparency and give it a number mark. This renders the idea manageable when collecting the data but can result in the lack of substance ethically. The concentration of those into one number may give an illusion of accuracy but obscure the argument of mutually opposed moral priorities. Some thinkers, such as Cartwright and Hardie suggest that thick modeling can be the best alternative that can reveal, as opposed to obscures, moral assumptions embedded in measurement. This entails the participation of the stakeholders, the contextualizing of indicators to the informed surroundings, and the possibility of the theoretical evaluative aspects of a concept to be discussed freely. This is in dramatic opposition to thin modeling that treats thick concepts as mostly fungible variables that can be interchanged in any dataset with no loss of meaning.

Composite Indicators and the Illusion of Neutrality

The possible best example of how normative decisions are obfuscated in technical design is found in composite indicators: indices that roll several variables into a single score. Health, education, and income are equally weighted in the HDI because the HDI itself decides to pick a normative representation of a world where the reduction of disparity will enhance societal happiness, and the HDI wants to be representative of this normative assumption. This would switch country rankings around dramatically were the weights altered and what is apparent objectivity is in fact not. As Sally Engle Merry (2011) notes, aggregation often masks internal tensions: a high education score might hide gender inequalities; a strong income score could obscure environmental degradation. Composite indicators seem to mask the multiplicity of human needs and values achieved by compressing a variety of dimensions into one number. James C. Scott (1998) calls this kind of simplification a "state simplification," a rendering of reality designed for administrative convenience rather than faithful representation. The ease of comparability and the immediate rankings by composite scores make them so tempting to policy-makers. Nevertheless, their attractiveness based on being simple is also what makes them ethically risky. The simplifying usage of a single upward trend line of the complex moral realities can give them a sense of complacency that ignores important aspects of injustice being difficult to see.

Indicators as Moral Gatekeepers

Indicators are moral gatekeepers since they determine what can be seen, measured, and acted on. They are not just mirrors that reflect the situation in the world; they inspire a direct influence upon it. Measures shape the priorities of governments, the use of resources at institutions, and the ways in which issues are brought into the public discourse. Martha Nussbaum (2013) warns against overreliance on GDP and similar growth-based metrics precisely because they crowd out other dimensions of human capability. When in a measurement, economic growth is valued more than capacity building or infrastructure provision more than people-engaged governance, then a hierarchy of morality is contained that elevates some forms of progress above other forms (Michalos & Hatch, 2020). The indicators serving as gatekeepers implies that inappropriate design of metrics might result in moral misdirection. The numerators count all the ways people participate in the company of others through activities based on community deliberation, or grassroots mobilization but these richer forms of democratic participation can be overlooked when measured in mere voter turnout. A focus on environmental performance means that a more holistic environmental picture in terms of biodiversity, cultural connection to the land, or environmental justice might be left out of policy considerations when carbon emissions are the only factor. In a nutshell, measurements are not merely neutral descriptions of things already out there; rather, they are used to generate the things that they help to create. They decide who can be seen, what is appreciated, and whose pain is recognized. Their neutral treatment is to overlook the normative architecture by which they are both endowed with meaning and invested with power.

The Politics of Visibility: What Metrics Reveal and Conceal

It is neither the ability to describe, but the possibility to speculate on what one can see and what is not to be seen, which makes the epistemic and normative power of metrics. Measurement tools used in the sphere of justice do not just represent reality; they create it. The technologies of this visibility, the technologies of that moral optic are signs, which constitute the visibility, the moral optic, within which such inequality, suffering, and injustice come into focus, or are in the shadows. This dual role means that metrics is not the passive image of social life but it serves as the determinant of parameters of recognition. The indicators define the limits of legibility by selecting what to measure and how. They allocate institutional concern to certain matters but not to others, preferring to act on them with policy measures. This partial enlightenment can never be neutral: It is at once an epistemic intervention and a political act. Relying on the theory of biopolitics posited by Michel Foucault, the description of symbolic violence proposed by Pierre Bourdieu, and critical studies of epistemology and ethics, this section analyzes the ways in which metrics may be used to both exert control and create divisions.

Foucault: Metrics, Biopolitics, and Governmentality

The concept of biopolitics developed by Michel Foucault provides one of the best ways to consider the political stakes of quantification. In his lectures at the Collège de France, Foucault (2008) describes biopolitics as the governance of life itself through the management of populations, achieved not by overt repression, but through technologies of normalization and surveillance. Statistics, benchmarks, and indicators are not mere neutral facts within such a framework because they are central tools of governmentality. Through such instruments, populations are categorized according to the degrees of risk, productivity, compliance, and health reshaping political questions into questions that appear technical. A justice measure of equality of opportunity, say, implicitly endorses a specific liberal ideal, and will make invisible other injustices like historical dispossession, structural violence, or collective trauma. By framing certain phenomena as measurable and others as irrelevant, metrics operate as what Foucault calls "dispositifs" (apparatuses) - structures that shape how we see, interpret, and act upon social realities. This is not just a process on metrics of justice, it goes through all the realms of health, education, and security. As Nikolas Rose (2009) observes, the governance of populations through indicators turns contested moral and political judgments into apparently objective, scientific facts. This shift in transformation restricts the area of political dialogue and centralizes powers in technocratic sort of authorities. This leads to depoliticization of justice, since the dispute over what is moral is pegged back as a technical disagreement about the design of measurements.

Bourdieu: Symbolic Violence and the Imposition of Norms

The theory of symbolic violence proposed by Pierre Bourdieu is a significant addition to the narrative proposed by Foucault as it helps to complement his writing by adding a cultural and epistemic layer to the issue of domination. The symbolic violence happens when the meanings and values of the dominant groups are enforced on others in the name of objectivity or universality. (Bourdieu, 1991). In metrics terms, this is usually along the lines of universalizing culturally specific norms and marginalizing or pathologizing other ways of knowing and valuing. This is evidently laid out in terms of global education indicators whereby the provision of quality education is determined, to a considerable degree, by the results of standardized tests. The result of such measures is the systematic devaluation of indigenous pedagogies, oral knowledge forms, relational learning, as something irrelevant or lacking in quality. This is not an accidental neglect; this is one aspect of the power structure where powerful epistemologies determine the existence of knowledge and competence. The realization that brings Bourdieu an insight is the fact that social hierarchies are encoded in apparently unbiased tools thanks to such processes. In this way, metrics may reinstate the epistemic domination by preconditioning the cognitive and cultural space, thus placing some groups of people in the limelight and making others invisible. Technical imposition of the norms by means of the indicators is not just that one, it is the form of the cultural power, which forms the basis of the question of the morality itself.

Metrics and Representational Injustice

Justice is more than distributional fairness and procedural equality justice; justice is also representation; it means being seen and treated as a number in the arrangements that determine how one lives. Nancy Fraser (2009) identifies misrepresentation and misrecognition as key forms of injustice, and these are directly implicated in the politics of metrics. When indicators fail to capture the realities of marginalized communities through conceptual omission, sampling bias, or interpretive erasure, they contribute to what Miranda Fricker (2007) terms hermeneutical injustice: the structural exclusion of certain groups from the processes of meaning-making. As an example, a gender justice measure consisting of binary gender categories will never reflect the gender-nonconforming nor the nonbinary subjects into the statistics, remaining invisible to statistical methods of measurement, thus not allowing their particular kind of vulnerability to be voiced. Equally, an aggregate indicator such as the Gini coefficient will record the degree of inequality, yet conceal its causes and distributions, raced based, caste based, geographically based, or disability based. This flattening strips away the ethical particularity of injustice, and displays it as a monolith (Michalos & Hatch, 2020).

In this way metrics become moral cartographies: they mark out the landscape of injustice in specifying what harms will or will not be charted. When the map excludes especially considerable injustices, the outcome is not that of simple carelessness but rather something where the over and over again reproduction of epistemic silencing occurs.

Moral Erasure Through Aggregation

Probably the most pernicious mode of invisibility in metrics is aggregation. Indicators provide simplifications of rather complex realities by smoothing down the range of measured data by averaging it or turning it into composite scores based on a combination of different data points. Much as this can help in terms of comparability and communication, it can lead to depoliticization of a reality of lived injustice. James C. Scott (1998), in *Seeing Like a State*, shows how "legibility" projects—designed to make societies administratively comprehensible, often erase the particularities that matter most to those who live within them. In the quest to be legible, aggregated indicators may erase a moral context: the fact that a national average has been improving may conceal an aggravating situation of disadvantaged subpopulations. Take an example in which the populace has increased average life expectancy and the native population is experiencing negative health gains. The overall figure is a sign of progress but the distribution behind the figure is an illustration of increasing inequality. In such cases, aggregation becomes an instrument of what Sylvia Wynter (2003) calls the "genre of Man": a statistical construct that normalizes the experiences of dominant groups while rendering others epistemologically absent. This is an ethical issue and not a technical one. Aggregation sends a speechless message that there are lives and sufferings, which are not deserving of being singled out in inquiry.

The politics of visibility warns that metrics are not only empirical tools but also moral and political tools. They determine who gets into the frame of recognition, whose sufferings can be read as legitimate by power, and what kinds of injustices can be negotiated in the realm of policy talk. Foucault warns how indicators can be used as technologies of governmental control; Bourdieu illustrates how they can impose cultural hegemony; and Fraser and Fricker explain how they can contribute to representational and hermeneutical injustice, whereas Wynter can show how aggregation can erase the lives it is supposed to represent. Recognizing these dynamics does not require abandoning metrics altogether. It demands that they be designed epistemically humbly, participatively, and normatively reflexively. The indicators are not just counting, but are to be made in a manner such that they shed a light, and are to be constructed in a manner that it is not easy to delete them, to give recognition to plural voices and to shed light over those lives and experiences most at risk of disappearing. It is through it that we are able to turn the politics of visibility not to become a way of injustice, but a way of righting a wrong.

Justice as a Meta-Norm: Can It Be an Indicator?

Justice holds an epistemically and normatively uncertain role in the context of social measurement. It is, on the one hand, a meta-norm, a criterion by which indicators validity, policies fairness, and the legitimacy of the institutional results are evaluated. On the other, it is becoming subject to greater entrapment into the world of operational measures, being converted into quantifiable elements within the social well-being systems and governance dashboards. This bidirectional position throws up a vexing query: can justice simultaneously be a meta-norm as well as a pointer without compromising its conceptual purity? Amartya Sen (2009) cautions against treating justice as a fully specifiable blueprint, instead framing it as a comparative practice that identifies and addresses "remediable injustices." According to this perspective, justice is not an object but a serious system of deliberation, the one that guides reflection on how institutions are to be designed, how they are to reason with each other, and how human beings ought to flourish. It is valuable because of its way of constructing inquiry rather than its ability to be reduced, into a score. As soon as justice is translated to quantitative language, its political and idealizing roles are at risk of being subsumed by administrative bureaucracy so it now becomes an issue of adherence rather than moral acting out. The tension here is not purely theoretical. The modern system of governance, which is under pressure to deliver hard measurements, tends to drag justice into the performance measurement range. The trick is to accomplish this, without removing from it the richness of its evaluation and its potency as political.

The Problem of Operationalization and the Risk of Reification

Contrary to philosophical reservations that have good reasons, the empirical call to get justice brought to measurable levels is high. Policy-makers and international bodies routinely employ proxies such as perceived fairness scores, legal access indices, or representation ratios—examples include the World Justice Project's Rule of Law Index. Although these tools can be heuristically useful, they are guilty to use a term of art in the discussion of moral conceptions, of what may be termed normative thinness. In a political-philosophical sense, justice is a multidimensional construct and contextual in that it cannot be reduced. Rawls (1971) foregrounds distributional fairness, Fraser (2003) emphasizes recognition, Nussbaum (2013) extends the concept to human capabilities, and Young (1990) insists on structural critique. It may indeed be questionable whether any attempt to minimize this breadth into a unitary measure of numerical invoice will not have the effect of compressing its content, at the cost of conceptual perforation into administrative comfort.

Even widely used proxies can mislead. Perceived fairness, for instance, may be skewed by ideological internalization: as Charles Mills (1997) observes in his critique of ideal theory, oppressed groups sometimes internalize unjust conditions as natural or deserved. In this situation, high scores of fairness may actually be an indicator of effective normalization of injustice and not the lack of it. The more profound philosophical danger is that of reification: the objectification of justice, by turning it into an inert object that includes telling evaluation. Nancy Cartwright and Jeremy Hardie (2015) warn that indicators often present themselves as neutral when in fact they are saturated with moral assumptions. This process resonates with Max Horkheimer and Theodor Adorno's (1944) description of the "administered world," where moral disputes are settled through bureaucratic calculation and statistical legitimacy. Reification does not simply make discourse that is normative one-dimensional; it transforms the political practice. As Jacques Rancière (2004) might put it, quantification can become part of the "police order," a system that integrates dissent into the logic of governance, converting radical demands into manageable performance gaps. It is by this means that the transformative potential of justice is controlled, coded, and sanitized to work within the institutional system.

Toward Hybrid Metrics and Informational Pluralism

Rejecting justice indicators altogether is neither practical nor desirable. Measurement has undeniable value for diagnosis, transparency, and accountability. Thus, the challenge becomes to design hybrid solutions to the problem by maintaining the relative luminosity of indicators and at the same time the normative density that the justice as meta-norm was supposed to capture. Sen's (1992) principle of "informational pluralism" provides a conceptual foundation for this approach. Rather than relying on a single metric or informational space, assessments should draw from multiple sources, each capturing different aspects of justice-relevant phenomena. This could mean combining the following:

- Quantitative data: Such as access rates, representation ratios, and funding disparities.
- Narrative accounts: Testimonies from affected communities, oral histories, and qualitative documentation of exclusion or dignity violations.
- Deliberative inputs: Participatory procedures in which the stakeholders review the legitimacy and equity.
- Contextual diagnostics: Analyses grounded in local histories, cultural frameworks, and structural conditions.

These hybrid models would not fall into the temptation of converting justice indicators into verdicts. However, they would act as catalysts to ethical thinking as jumping off points of disagreement, not arrival points of adjudication. In line with Sally Engle Merry's (2011) insistence on contestability, indicators would be explicitly provisional, open to revision, and embedded in democratic deliberation.

This reconfiguration also mitigates the dangers of reification. Indicators can no longer so easily pass by posing as complete or self-sufficient accounts of justice when tied to narratives, participatory processes, and implications of contextual interpretation. Their part becomes that of the voice of moral authority instead of a statement on moral authority. Finally, justice is perhaps best thought of in terms other than as a measurable object, but as what could be called a regulative ideal: a horizon that cannot be closed or brought to rest against which one continues to reflect ethically. Indicators can and should be used, but only in circumstances where they form part of a framework that takes account of their biased, perspective-driven nature. It is not the desire to render justice legible to statistics in its totality but rather to clarify its absences and distortion as well as its potentials using statistics. Justice indicators in this sense are most philosophically defensible when they are indicators that do not want to be and cannot be definitive, when they manifest the limits of their blind spots, when they draw our attention away toward other directions. Thoughtfully constructed, hybrid measures have the potential to promote justice, but not at the expense of justice, a culture of moral imagination not a technocratic end game.

Pluralism, Contestability, and Democratic Design

Whatever measure to gauge justice professes itself to do so is of moral resolute and consequently subjected to challenge. The situation of contestability is not a design flaw, it is a protection against epistemic closure and normative authoritarianism. There is a danger that an indubitable measure of justice may become like a weapon rather than a means of inclusion because it drowns out other moral viewpoints and auto-justification. Sally Engle Merry (2011), in her critique of human rights indicators, underscores that metrics "encode values, prioritize goals, and shape social realities." Unless such values and priorities are impossible to challenge, indicators may pose a threat of becoming a means of hegemony instead of justice. In order to be treated as legitimate in the democratic process they must be subject to challenge, reinterpretation, and denial. Philosophically, contestability goes with the epistemic humility that is needed in value pluralism. Isaiah Berlin (1969) argued that there are multiple, legitimate, and incommensurable conceptions of the good, none of which can be fully subsumed under a single metric. Elizabeth Anderson (1993) similarly maintains that justice must allow for reasonable moral disagreement. Against this backdrop of a thought experiment, justice measures have to be structured to permit such disagreement, so that in addition to technical adjustment, there is normative reconsideration of what to measure, how to measure, and why to measure.

Democratic Legitimacy and the Co-Construction of Metrics

The authority of the creation of these metrics endows them with normative power not only in the accuracy of their statistical compilation but also in the legitimacy of their production. Amartya Sen (2009) emphasizes that social indicators should be rooted in public reasoning, a deliberative process through which citizens collectively examine, debate, and refine the criteria of justice (Maurya, 2021). Not a procedural afterthought, this is a principal requirement of ethical measurement. Nancy Fraser's (2003) principle of participatory parity strengthens this claim. Fraser adds the aspect of participation in the decisions on how justice will be judged; this, he believes justice needs in addition to fair distribution and cultural recognition. Such inclusion is necessary, as without it even metrics developed technically will reproduce structural exclusion. Boaventura de Sousa Santos (2014) takes this further, calling for "epistemologies of the South" to dismantle the monopoly of dominant knowledge systems in indicator design. Communities too long historically relegated to the sideline as mere objects of knowledge production must have equal epistemic weight in determining what and how we measure in postcolonial contexts particularly.

Participatory Approaches: Deliberation, Narrative, Experience

The participatory styles of engagement change the epistemic position of the measured ones, as the passive targets of data into the active source of ability with regard to justice-relevant data. They question embedded belief that what has legitimacy is statistical wise method mediated by experts. Miranda Fricker's (2007) concept of epistemic injustice is crucial here. She also determines that marginalized communities experience credibility loss and are unable to affect formal system of knowledge with their ideas. Applied to measurement, this implies that the groups most vulnerable to injustice tend to bear the least control over how it is structured, categorized, and handled. This has been attempted to be redressed by participatory processes that seek redistribution of hermeneutical power, where those who suffer injustice would also design the conceptual and methodological terms of its measurement. Concrete participatory methods include:

- Deliberative forums: Group meetings where people collectively nominate justice concerns and jointly draft measures.
- Narrative inquiry: The incorporation of tales of rejection, survival, and renewal into the conceptual weft of indicators.
- Experiential surveys: These were used to measure affective, symbolic, and relational aspects of justice, including dignity, recognition, and procedural fairness.

These approaches embody a pluralistic epistemology. They reject a quantitative instrumentalism of completely disembodied accounts of justice through demanding that the lived, contextual accounts are essential to a proper understanding of justice. They also resonate with Martha Nussbaum's (2013) capabilities framework, which emphasizes dignity and agency as nonnegotiable elements of any evaluation of human well-being.

Reflexivity and Ethical Responsiveness

Design inclusivity should be accompanied by application reflexivity. Reflexivity is understood to imply a self-regulatory ethical wariness of assumptions and omissions and the implications of measurement. Indicators cannot be considered neutral observers that reflect on social reality the way it is, but rather interpretive mediations, and as such they should be approached. Nancy Cartwright and Jeremy Hardie (2015) argue that the best policy tools are not those that claim neutrality, but those that acknowledge their value-laden nature and remain open to critique. The acceptance of revision in reflexive indicators is not an option, but encouraged, with a view that metrics are living tools as opposed to pronouncement. This kind of reflexivity requires meta-ethical position: the acknowledgment that the indicators are never full-blown, final, and in unproblematic locales of moral terrain. In the absence of it even the indicators of participatory and inclusive can become the instruments of epistemic closure. The justice indicators are not to be merely statistically valid or methodologically sound. They must be epistemically both plural and reflexive as well as democratically legitimate. The aspect of contestability is not to be regarded as a design risk but as structural protection. Participatory design can legitimately be seen not only as good practice but as a moral requirement of any action purporting to embody justice. Pluralism guarantees that there is a lack of a single worldview monopolizing the meaning of justice. Contestability keeps moral debate alive. Democratic design gives more power to those most affected to design their own tools that will embody their realities. Reflexivity prevents metrics from solidifying into tools of domination. In combination, these principles indicate a democratic ethic of measurement, a context where justice is not instrumentalized into a number but rather explored and, in the collaborative spirit, a joint and ongoing horizon of ethical pursuit. The points in this model would not provide the definitive answer, but would rather be invitations to joint thinking, continuous criticism, and moral imagination.

Justice Beyond Measurement: Alternative Ethico-Political Paradigms

The Limits of Quantification: Questioning the Epistemic Empire

In the present, the current obsession with quantification at the state level (the form of which is indicators, audits, and ranking among nations) has completely transformed how people conceive and seek justice. Although it can be said that metrics can throw light on patterns of inequality and allow cross-sectionality of comparison, not all injustices can be measured and not all measurements are proportionate to the moral weight that they purport to reflect. Martha Nussbaum (2013) acknowledges that even within the capabilities approach, a framework that aspires to combine normative depth with operational clarity, there remain domains where "narrative and testimony" may be ethically superior to aggregated data. Similarly, Sally Engle Merry (2016) warns that the global proliferation of governance-by-indicators reflects a broader audit culture that displaces democratic deliberation with technocratic evaluation, privileging managerial logic over human need. What it produces is what is largely called a creeping epistemic empire, and the measurable can obscure the meaningful.

Justice Without Metrics: Ethics of Care, Recognition, and Testimony

Is justice possible without quantification? The theory of competing ethics has its arguments on the affirmative, in fact, it states that when justice is translated into numerical measures, then it becomes inevitable that such measures obscure its very essential levels. The ethics of care, articulated by Carol Gilligan (1982) and expanded by Joan Tronto (1993), locates justice in attentiveness, relational responsibility, and responsiveness to need, qualities that resist quantification. Likewise, Iris Marion Young (1990) frames justice as communicative openness to marginalized voices, where testimony functions not as data but as an ethical encounter that compels acknowledgment and action (Maurya, 2020). These approaches resist the flattening effects of abstraction. They demand that justice exists, has being and historicity, and that its most pressing forms can be articulated in terms of narrations, memory, and practice instead of statistical form.

Critique of Indicator-Centric Governance

There has been a technocratic orientation in policy-making alongside the emergence of indicators as lingua franca of governance. As Michael Power (1997) describes in *The Audit Society*, institutions increasingly define success through measurable outputs, turning evaluation into a ritual detached from substantive ethical engagement.

This drift carries at least three risks:

- Technocracy: Numbers usurp the democratic logic in favor of expert bureaucracies.
- Surveillance: Indicators become instruments of population control, echoing Michel Foucault's (2008) critique of biopolitics and the "governmentalization of the state."
- Depoliticization: The problem of injustice is defined in technical rather than structural terms, dampening calls to transform the situation into adjustments in specific policies.

Within these regimes, measurements can overshadow the political interests of justice by redesigning it as a policy option, a neutral lever, and neutralizing the citizens moral agency.

Justice as Praxis: Responsiveness, Repair, and Historical Consciousness

Cornel West (2005) famously declared that "justice is what love looks like in public." The vision redefines justice as a practice rather than as a fixed result, that is, justice as praxis, justice as an ethical response to the lived reality of responsiveness, repair, and historic memory. Responsiveness prioritizes ethical proximity over statistical accountability (Kittay, 2019). Repair addresses historical injustices such as slavery, colonialism, and dispossession through acts of acknowledgment, restitution, and structural redress—not by simply quantifying their legacies. Historical consciousness would not allow past violence to be washed away in aggregation in the present, would demand that justice might be not a linear event but variously contextual and memory-bearing. Within this context the attempt to reductively convert justice into a value that itself acts as the indicator risks removing the harms and injury that provoked the need of justice, rendering moral practice disconnected from the history that is imbued with meaning.

Radical Traditions: Ethics Without Quantification

Traditions of decolonial, abolitionist, and feminist thought express, perhaps, the starkest challenge to the priorities of a measure-based justice. Boaventura de Sousa Santos (2014) calls for epistemologies of the South to counter the monoculture of scientific knowledge. These structures reject the common capture by indicators, claiming the side of pluriversal ways of knowledge and valuation. In the abolitionist tradition, Angela Davis (2003) and Ruth Wilson Gilmore (2007) envision justice not as reform within existing systems but as their transformation or dismantling. The ethical vision of a world in the absence of prisons cannot be grasped by, say, prison replace "reform" indicators. Black feminist thinkers center justice in lived resistance, relational solidarity, and intergenerational healing, domains where quantification is neither adequate nor desirable. These traditions do not depend on the assumption that justice should be readable to the states, markets, or donors. The performance of justice, to them, is practiced in community, struggle, and mutual care—something beyond the epistemic capability of dashboards and indices.

An attempt to critique the reign of the measurement is not to forfeit rationality or responsibility. It is not to claim rather the moral and political depth of justice as a relational but a historical, imaginative venture. Unmeasurable justice is not chaos: it signifies tending to such ethical realities as resist reduction, such as bereavement, solidarity, betrayal, and hope. The thing is not how the tools may be perfected then but whether some kinds of justice can or should not be administered in a quantifiable form at all. The injustices are such that they need not more precise indicators but worse kinds of listening, remembering, and acting. By fixing justice to what can be entirely counted we incur the risk of forgetting what remains unanswered.

Philosophical Guidelines for Ethical Justice Metrics

The normative commitments that dictate ethically robust justice metrics are supposed to be more than technically sufficient. These promises at least entail transparency, pluralism, inclusiveness, and epistemic humility. Transparency does not imply simply unveiled access to information, but a recognition of trade-offs and trade-offs that tended to be built into the process of constructing the indicators (Maurya, 2022). As Nancy Cartwright and Jeremy Hardie (2015) argue, indicators are "thick" with values and should never be presented as neutral mirrors of reality. Pluralism recognizes the irreducibility of justice to a single metric; drawing on Isaiah Berlin's (1969) value pluralism, it resists the temptation to impose a homogenized definition of the good life, allowing for coexisting and potentially conflicting justice claims. Inclusiveness demands the active participation of historically marginalized groups in defining and validating what justice means in measurable terms, aligning with Nancy Fraser's (2003) insistence on "participatory parity" as a normative condition of justice. Humility tempers the epistemic ambition of metrics with recognition of their inherent limitations, echoing Amartya Sen's (2009) reminder that justice is a comparative, context-sensitive concept, not a final blueprint to be encoded in indicators (Maurya, 2024).

The main ethical issue is the instrumentalization of justice metrics, i.e., reducing justice to management instrument or PR. In audit cultures (Power, 1997), indicators are often deployed to signal legitimacy rather than to drive structural transformation, severing the metric from its moral content and turning it into an administrative artifact devoid of critical power. Martha Nussbaum (2013) warns against the "technocratic drift" of well-being indicators, urging policy-makers to remember that justice is not a problem to be solved, but a normative orientation to be lived and continually revised. In circumstances whereby metrics are utilized to achieve institutional performance, instead of moral responsibility, they end up compromised morally. The metrics of ethical justice should thus be bound to governance-as-responsibility instead of governance-as-efficiency; the measure is not a maximization but a morally radical bearing.

The justice indicators should also be ingrained into the grander philosophical discussions of moral thinking and they cannot work in solipsism. This must be understood in terms of contextual moral insights, grounded in publicly reasoned justification, as opposed to statistical correlation, and as aimed at moral purposes, as opposed to technical objectives. Sen's (2009) model of public reasoning captures this approach, understanding justice through social dialogue and evaluative plurality, while Elizabeth Anderson (1993) emphasizes moral learning and contextual judgment in ethical evaluation—capacities that cannot be outsourced to algorithms or statistical models. In this sense metrics are morally powerful only when they are elements within a living discourse of ethics, understood not primarily as answers but rather as agitations to further questioning.

Lastly, indicators should not serve as epistemic verdicts, but must instead invite collective determination of the moral matters. They ought to demand thinking, objection, and moral imagination, rather than provide closure. As Sally Engle Merry (2016) observes, indicators are performative: they shape what is seen, valued, and acted upon. This performativity should be utilized in an ethical rather than foreclosing practice so as to infuse democratic conversation on the main meaning of justice. The indicators must make apparent their provisional, tentative nature, be subject to criticism and revision, and they must be conducted with dialogical processes that require several perspectives, histories, and moral vocabularies. By so doing, they are participants in bringing justice into view as a process, one that is inclusive and reflexive rather than a technocratic final fix.

At a time when measurements are continuing to dominate our institutional and moral existence, the philosophical role of measuring has never been so pressing. The metrics of justice should be established with ethical rules focusing on the moral depth, epistemic inclusivity, and democracy integrity. These guidelines have served as a reminder that justice is not a figure but has become a shared hope, a complicated aspirational goal, which is being constantly reinvented. Measurements can, and maybe will, help us in this effort, but only insofar as we use them as ethical tools, never as a means of reducing the content of, and limiting access to, the area of public reason, political accountability, and moral criticism.

Conclusion

The problem of quantifying justice constantly faces a painful philosophical paradox: how do you operationalize that which is normatively complex and ethically contentious and contextually tricky into numerically manipulable indicators? The notion of justice, as a moral ideal, is rife with quality, semantic variety, and indeterminate uber-aspirations. To quantify it is to render empty its content in the name of empirical accuracy. As Charles Taylor (1985) reminds us, ethical life is grounded in strong evaluations, value commitments that resist simple instrumental equivalence. The normative fabric of justice; its claims of dignity, recognition, suffering, and responsibility; transcend the scope of algorithmic presence. Measurement should thus be undertaken with a heightened sense of its boundaries, its metaphysical danger, and its threat to moral oblivion. The hazard has less to do with measure than with a certain epistemic reversal, in which measurements come to define and not serve justice (Maurya, 2025). Indicators have led to a transfer of normative power out of the hands of democratic communities into those of technocratic systems, where justice takes on a numerical value, representing the score, embodying the ranking, or as a benchmark. Martha Nussbaum (2013) makes this clear in Creating Capabilities: metrics can help track progress toward moral ends, but they cannot replace the critical, dialogical, and historically responsive work of defining those ends. Likewise, Amartya Sen (2009) insists that justice must remain grounded in public reasoning, an inclusive process of reflective scrutiny in which indicators participate, but never dominate.

It is the responsibility of philosophy to give up the open-ended work of moral judgment, handing it over to the closed system of algorithmic rationality, so as to permit metrics to constitute justice. By their nature, administration systems enhance simplicity, standardization, and surveillance, trends that are hardly neutral in morality. As James C. Scott (1998) documents in Seeing Like a State, technocratic simplifications often enact epistemic violence, erasing local knowledge, lived experience, and intricate social interdependencies in favor of abstractions legible only to centralized authorities. With the chapter ending and the book progressing to its closing reflection in Chap. 8 Toward a Just Society: Indicators to the Future, it is time to reconceive indicators not as reflections of moral fact but of ethical aspiration. Indicators must not serve to diminish justice but to point to it, to accept that it is complex, and to invite participatory clarification and development. Measuring justice is treading a philosophical tightrope: between ethical breadth and empirical generalization, populist participation, and bureaucratic codification. Yet the task is not hopeless. When embraced with humility, inclusivity, and reflexivity, justice metrics can clarify directions to existent moral development as a society. Ultimately, the question is not what measure of justice do we have, but how to measure that measure of justice in a just way.

References

Anderson, E. (1993). *Value in ethics and economics*. Harvard University Press.

Berlin, I. (1969). *Four essays on liberty*. Oxford University Press.

Bourdieu, P. (1991). *Language and symbolic power*. Harvard University Press.

Cartwright, N., & Hardie, J. (2015). *Evidence-based policy: A practical guide to doing it better*. Oxford University Press.

Davis, A. Y. (2003). *Are Prisons Obsolete?* Seven Stories Press.

Foucault, M. (1978). *The history of sexuality, volume 1: An introduction*. Vintage.

Fricker, M. (2007). *Epistemic injustice: Power and the ethics of knowing*. Oxford University Press.

Gilmore, R. W. (2007). *Golden gulag: Prisons, surplus, crisis, and opposition in globalizing California*. University of California Press.

Habermas, J. (1987). *The theory of communicative action* (Vol. II). Beacon Press.

Harding, S. (1992). Rethinking standpoint epistemology: What is "Strong Objectivity"? In L. Alcoff & E. Potter (Eds.), *Feminist epistemologies*. Routledge.

Kant, I. (1785/1996). Groundwork for the metaphysics of morals (trans. Mary Gregor). Cambridge University Press.

Kittay, E. F. (2019). *Love's labor: Essays on women, equality and dependency*. Routledge.

Michalos, A. C., & Hatch, P. M. (2020). Good societies, financial inequality and secrecy, and a good life: From Aristotle to Piketty. *Applied Research in Quality of Life, 15*(3), 1005–1054. https://doi.org/10.1007/s11482-019-09717-0

Longino, H. (1990). *Science as social knowledge: Values and objectivity in scientific inquiry*. Princeton University Press.

Merry, S. E. (2011). Measuring the world: Indicators, human rights, and global governance. *Current Anthropology, 52*(S3), S83–S95.

Maurya, S. K. (2025). Restorative justice and karmic justice: Ubuntu and Vedanta in dialogue. *African Journal of Religion, Philosophy and Culture, 6*(2).

Maurya, S. K. (2024). African philosophies of justice and equity: A contemporary discourse. *African Journal of Religion, Philosophy and Culture, 5*(2), 61–78. https://doi.org/10.31920/2634-7644/2024/v5n2a4

Maurya, S. K. (2022). On just, justice and distributive justice: A critical and comparative discourse. *Journal of Liberty and International Affairs, 8*(2), 240–254. https://doi.org/10.47305/JLIA2282240m

Maurya, S. K. (2021). The concept of justice in reference with philosophies of Plato and Aristotle: A critical study. *Journal of Liberty and International Affairs, 7*(3), 250–266. https://doi.org/10.47305/JLIA21370250m

Maurya, S. K. (2020). A reply to Louis P. Pojman's article "The case against affirmative action". *Conatus—Journal of Philosophy, 5*(2), 87–113.

Merry, S. E. (2016). *The seductions of quantification: Measuring human rights, gender violence, and sex trafficking*. University of Chicago Press.

Mills, C. W. (1997). *The racial contract*. Cornell University Press.

Nussbaum, M. C. (2013). *Creating capabilities: The human development approach*. Harvard University Press.

Porter, T. M. (2020). *Trust in numbers: The pursuit of objectivity in science and public life*. Princeton University Press.

Power, M. (1997). *The audit society: Rituals of verification*. Oxford University Press.

Rancière, J. (2004). *Disagreement: Politics and philosophy*. University of Minnesota Press.

Rawls, J. (1971). *A theory of justice*. Harvard University Press.

Rose, N. (2009). *Powers of freedom: Reframing political thought*. Cambridge University Press.

Santos, B. d. S. (2014). *Epistemologies of the south: Justice against epistemicide*. Routledge.

Scott, J. C. (1998). *Seeing like a state: How certain schemes to improve the human condition have failed*. Yale University Press.

Sen, A. (1992). *Inequality reexamined*. Harvard University Press.

Sen, A. (2009). *The idea of justice*. Harvard University Press.

West, C. (2005). *Democracy matters: Winning the fight against imperialism*. Penguin.

Wynter, S. (2003). Unsettling the coloniality of being/power/truth/freedom. *CR: The New Centennial Review, 3*(3), 257–337.

Chapter 8
Toward a Just Society: Indicators for the Future

Introduction: The Future of Justice as a Measurable Ideal

The desire to quantify justice, is a the complex task that has been considered in the past as one filled with knowledge doubts and more ethical questions than answers, would require a radical philosophical rethinking when extended into the future. Traditionally an ideal of moral and political thought, Justice is entering the technocratic worlds of measures, evaluation, and control. It is this change of norm to number that requires our critical questioning not only of what we count, but of what our counting is doing to this very idea of justice itself. This final chapter defends a normative philosophy of justice, a philosophy in which justice is not a perfected state of morals, nor a kind of equilibrium within institutions, but a morally inspired ideal of the future intrinsic to the civic imagination, the reasoning of the public, and the future-oriented policy-making. Justice is not fully achieved in the present; hence, it is the lack of complete realization in the present that makes it normatively urgent to ask the question of how we should envisage and assess justice in the future. Justice as an ideal that can be measured should not degenerate into a fact administered; justice should always be pegged to our collective moral panorama.

The classical tradition and much of it later, including Plato in *The Republic* and Kant in *The Metaphysics of Morals*, had considered justice as a transcendent, never wholly explicable, and always theoretically linked to harmony, self-rule, or dispassion. Yet, as Amartya Sen (2009) argues in *The Idea of Justice*, we need a shift from transcendental institutionalism to a comparative, realization-oriented framework, one sensitive to plural values, contextual injustice, and the possibility of greater rather than perfect justice. This reconfiguration places justice as a moving and future-oriented evaluative orientation rather than a state reached and frozen in time. Then justice is something we have out to the future rather than looking back on it upon established principles. This opens a space for richer engagement with ethical imagination, anticipatory governance (Guston, 2014), and critical-utopian

S. K. Maurya, *Exploring Justice as a Social Indicator of Life*, Social Indicators Research Series 92, https://doi.org/10.1007/978-3-032-10812-8_8

thinking (Levitas, 2013), where imagining justice futures becomes a moral task in itself.

Indicators as Generative, Not Merely Reflective, Tools

Traditional descriptions portray social indicators as a means of explaining an existing reality, the statistical picture of the prevailing distribution of goods, harms, or rights. But this is reductive understanding of the same. As scholars of social constructivism have long emphasized, indicators are not merely mirrors; they are scripts (Merry, 2016). They consume the world they claim to quantify by fashioning the world through performance of measurement that changes the way we think, behave, distribute resources, and gauge value. Metrics, in this light, are technologies of world-making. They determine what can be seen, what issues are considered as urgent, and whose life should be respected. Justice indicators are thus never ethically neutral, they are value-laden instruments encoding political priorities, institutional norms, and philosophical commitments. The design of them is not only a technical task but a good and an ethical issue. Future instruments should not simply be judged in terms of their methodological soundness but also in terms of their moral generativity: Do they serve to make societies more just by aiding in reflection, opening up, and criticism? Or are they preemptive of reasoning, purporting to present an illusion of finality and exactness?

Some philosophical courage is required to imagine various ways in which criminal justice in the future might be signaled by the future, a boldness to transcend the inherited categories, path dependencies of institutions, and bureaucratic expediency. As Charles Taylor (2004) has argued, modernity suffers from an "immanent frame," a constriction of imagination that resists transcendence and moral possibility. What is needed to break such a frame is normative plurality and principled normative clarity. Such clarity does not entail consensus or simplification. On the contrary, it requires attending to contested values, epistemic pluralism, and the moral complexity of lived experiences. For instance, indicators of justice must balance recognitional concerns (Fraser, 2008), capabilities for agency (Nussbaum, 2011), and ecological sustainability, a task that demands ethical coherence alongside contextual flexibility. This is not an easy task. It entails maneuvering between the Scylla of the normative vagueness in which metrics lose their moral capacity to relate as they are morally sterile and the Charybdis of the dogmatic formalism spoken of above that results in the reification of one rather narrow vision of justice at the cost of all others.

Going forward on the future of justice indicators, the question is not whether we measure justice, measurement is here to stay, but how we do it in a manner that respects the moral depth, ontological plurality, and political contestability of the concept itself. Indicators should not be taken as destinations but as moral proposals; tentative means in our shared task of living together in a world that is mired in structural injustice, past traumas, and democratic dreams. The challenge before us is to make sure our indicators do not limit our moral imagination but instead shine a light around the routes to the justice that is never finished, but always being made.

Normative Criteria for Future Justice Indicators

The justice-based indicator design is not a technical activity but a moral one. The indicators are not just data instruments, but normative tools of judgment. As Amartya Sen (2009) emphasizes, they inevitably reflect and reproduce specific moral visions of the good life, fairness, and legitimacy. Moreover, the future of justice metric frameworks should hence be based on healthy normative ideas as a compromise between empirical relatability and philosophical richness. These four interdependent principles, namely, inclusiveness, pluralism, flexibility, and moral transparency provide a guideline on how to make the measurement of justice ethically responsible. The inclusion principle would claim that indicators must offset the marginalized not merely within the measurement range of the data but within the epistemic framework of the measure itself. This includes making sure that the worldviews, values, and vocabularies of historically excluded groups feature into the actual structure of indicators themselves. As Nancy Fraser (2008) argues, justice entails not only redistribution but recognition and participatory parity. In this context, inclusiveness means acknowledging the hermeneutic agency of marginalized communities (Fricker, 2007) by asking who defines justice, whose suffering is statistically visible, and who is epistemically authorized to speak. Examples abound: indicators of educational justice should address not only enrollment rates but the lived experiences of racialized, disabled, or indigenous students often excluded from standard frameworks (Santos, 2014). Gender equity policies must also do away with binary classifications to include the intersectional lives of trans, queer, and nonbinary persons. This all-inclusiveness can be engendered only in the form of dialogical not extractive processes, in response to the call of Boaventura de Sousa Santos to explore, also, the notion of epistemologies of the South, which envisage epistemic justice as part shouldering the inquiry into justice itself, rather than a joint periphery.

The second principle, pluralism, implies that indicators must accept moral and cultural diversity. Isaiah Berlin's (1969) concept of value pluralism, wherein distinct, often incommensurable values may all be valid, applies directly to metric design. Justice in a plural world cannot be reduced to a scalar measure, or an objective score. Rather, it must be multidimensional, capable of accepting conflicting/competing values like freedom, equality, dignity, solidarity, and sustainability. This pluralism also has to be accommodative of competing ontologies of justice: in one society, justice is predicated upon balance and returns; in another, it is predicated upon relationality or harmony with nature or cross-generational stewardship. In the absence of such institutionalizing of pluralism as a design principle, such culturally situated understandings will continue to be absent in formal systems of measurement.

Flexibility is equally crucial. Justice is historically accountable, politically contentious, and environmentally responsive, making the measures that endeavor to express it adaptable according to societal development. Rigid indicators risk obsolescence, or worse, perpetuating injustice. Early versions of the Human Development Index (HDI), for instance, overlooked intragroup disparities, ecological degradation, and subjective well-being, all now recognized as central to justice discourse. This flexibility is not arbitrariness but flexibility to include new dimensions as new kinds of exclusion or injustice become possible, whether in algorithmic bias or displacement-driven climate change. This kind of flexibility will depend upon institutional reflexivity, that is, the existence of a process of periodic reevaluation, contestation, and democratic revamping that would guarantee that, justice measures are morally consistent and remain socially significant.

Finally, moral transparency is indispensable. Each indicator of justice has value judgments about which results count, which groups should be emphasized, which trade-offs are acceptable. These are "thick" ethical assumptions, yet they are often obscured behind a veneer of objectivity. This "illusion of neutrality" (Merry, 2016) facilitates technocratic drift, transforming justice into a matter of technical optimization rather than public moral reasoning. To resist this, indicators should spell out their normative assumptions: why specific variables are used, the values they convey, whose interests to whom, and which are their moral theories of being, be it capabilities-based, needs-based, or rights-based. This kind of transparency will lead to improved accountability and civic education where the metrics are transformed into ethical teachings that enable citizens to define and develop their own intuitions about justice.

These features of inclusiveness, pluralism, flexibility, and transparency are thus not adjuncts but prerequisites to any measure of justice that merits that designation. In their absence, metrics can cause justice to be narrowed down to bureaucratic performance or numerical abstraction. On the basis of these principles, however, indicators can become an ethical toolbox, they can make the invisible visible, they can make the moral imagination work, and they can ground governance in public reason. The parliaments and the street protests will be abandoned, and the future of justice will be determined in those silent spaces of the measurement architecture where the ethical pledges behind our indicators will allow us to determine the moral vistas in which society will attempt to aim in the direction of accommodation marked.

Anticipatory Governance and the Ethics of Forecasting

To preserve its moral relevance in a world undergoing a swift transformation, justice must no longer be locked into the backward-looking business of adjudicating on past wrongs. It should also be a forward-looking normative compass to act in a state of uncertainty, emergence, and interdependence. The design of future justice indicators therefore cannot rest solely on historical trend-lines or static benchmarks; it must embrace anticipatory governance, the normative practice of governing through informed foresight (Guston, 2014). These indicators are not neutral gauges of some reality out there; as a material of time, they shape the set of possible futures that societies see around them as possible or desirable and conceal others. They have the power to inform the ways governments, institutions, and citizens imagine what justice across time should entail through their embeddedness in specific assumptions regarding causality, agency, and temporal responsibility.

The normative stakes of predictive indicators are considerable. Social unrest early warnings and climate risk forecasts or algorithmic fairness ratings are meant to predict justice-related conditions, yet forecasting is never normatively non-oppressive in itself. It poses very profound normative doubts regarding probabilism, moral responsibility, and human agency. As Sheila Jasanoff (2010) argues in her account of "sociotechnical imaginaries," collectively held visions of desirable futures are stabilized through technology and governance, often acquiring a taken-for-granted authority. Such imaginaries can be internalized within institutions of practice by the functionalities of predictive indicators, locking in unidimensional conceptions of what justice is and maintaining what is dubbed as the insemination of narrow imaginaries, preempting dissent or marginalizing others. However, to give a specific example, a justice metric based on linear increases in educational equity may push into the background more radical or community-centric pedagogical functions that lie outside of its frame of measurement. Theoretically, in these instances predictive measures become self-fulfilling prophecies, with interventions being driven by bureaucratic stagnation and technical path-dependence more than the open, democratic process.

Avoiding this form of metric determinism requires cultivating what has been called futures literacy—the capacity to imagine, assess, and deliberate upon multiple, ethically distinct futures (Miller, 2018). The important thing about futures literacy is it is not about getting the single answer; it is about enlarging the moral and political horizon of possibility. Mathematically speaking, measures of justice ought to facilitate moral imagination and not limit it. They must invite contestation, plural reflection, and deliberative refinement. Martha Nussbaum (2011) underscores that justice requires narrative sensitivity: the capacity to apprehend and engage with the situated aspirations, vulnerabilities, and capabilities of others across time. Draped in these terms, forecasting is less a calling to soothsay what will occur and more an incitement, an opening to civic consideration of long-term advantage, intergenerational duty, and the ethical texture of future worlds.

Moral responsibility in the future is also brought into high relief by anticipatory justice metrics. Whose suffering is anticipated and addressed? Whose lives are imagined as worth protecting? The risks, whose visibility in the frame of calculation have been made or not? Hans Jonas argued that modern technological power generates an unprecedented ethical duty: not only to avoid foreseeable harm but to preserve the preconditions for human flourishing far into the future (Jonas, 1984). Indicators that do not consider emerging harms, such as those caused by climate collapse, algorithmic discrimination, ecological degradation, or intergenerational indebtedness, lack not only breadth, but a moral content.

To this extent, justice measures in the future must incorporate what we can term moral temporality: the recognition that the present has obligations to future generations, to communities that have been unheard, and the dispossessed due to something like environmental change or political dispossession. It is an ethic of time that opposes the moral minimalism, i.e., the moral philosophy in which the future harms will not matter as much, and the linear extrapolation, according to which tomorrow will just be an expansion of today. Rather, it demands the elaboration of signals capable of responding to changing contexts, revealing underrepresented dangers, and motivating democratic induction into potential futures. Such an approach reconfigures the role of indicators themselves. They are no longer fixed images of present reality, but are transformed into ethical world-making instruments. The indicators of this paradigm are not closure-gadgets, which pronounce the state of justice a settled matter; they are discursive portals-openings into the account of what justice might and ought to be in the years and decades to come. This is anticipatory governance in a nutshell: it is not the matter of being ready to expect likely happenings, but rather the morality of being receptive to futures we have yet to learn to dream about.

In this respect, the construction and application of future-oriented indicators of justice require philosophical boldness. They have to resist the lure of small technocratic rationality and accept the disunity included in moral life. These should be pluralist, reflexive, as well as inclusive as envisaged in democratic processes that hold them open to contestation. Most importantly, they need to consider justice as a potentially shifting future horizon; it is something that needs dynamic generation over time spanned across generations, not appraisal. When taken in this spirit, anticipatory governance has the power to transform indicators into living moral provocations that can guide societies toward not only the future that they can anticipate, but also the future that they have not yet dreamed.

Global Justice and Post-Western Epistemologies

The call to global justice initiatives creates interventions to geopolitical configuration in a geographic location significant as to the extent of epistemic asymmetry. Dominant measurement systems, whether GDP, the Human Development Index (HDI), or the Sustainable Development Goals (SDGs), are largely products of Euro-Atlantic knowledge regimes, and thus often fail to recognize, let alone integrate, diverse ontologies of justice, well-being, and relationality. As Santos (2014) observes, what is presented as "universal" knowledge is frequently "abyssal": it draws an invisible line that relegates non-Western epistemologies to the realm of the irrelevant or nonexistent. In these circumstances, achieving global justice is not merely an affair of adding measurements of the Global South to established schemes. Instead, it must involve a fundamentally radical decolonization of the epistemological premise that informs justice measurement, an endeavor based on cognitive justice, epistemic plurality, and relational responsibility.

The vision offered by Boaventura de Sousa Santos of the need to practice epistemologies of the South highlights the fact that justice should be perceived in light of the existence of other knowledges, that is, of understandings that are contoured around indigenous, subaltern, and non-Western worldviews. Cognitive justice would not only involve realization of fair material results, but the epistemic parity: the right of other systems of knowledge to determine the conditions of justice on their own. This new orientation requires a task of disengagement with the rhetoric of universalism or what Santos has termed (the pluriverse) that there are many worlds and consequently many possible measures. For example, in Andean cosmology, the principle of sumak kawsay (often translated as "good living") privileges harmony with nature, reciprocity within community, and the maintenance of ecological balance over the pursuit of individual autonomy or material consumption. These values are not measured in most of the Western-made indicators of development and well-being that specifically reward productivity, income, and consumption as being major indicators of progress. To be just, global justice indicators must speak across epistemic borders, and even in a conceptual sense they must be multilingual. In turn, this necessitates codesign processes whereby the marginalized groups are no longer mere participants in surveys, but vocal participants in the development of the conceptual categories as well as the normative assumptions around which the metrics are developed.

The ineffectiveness of common indicator systems is further brought to light by indigenous views on justice. As Whyte (2018) explains, many indigenous traditions conceive of justice in relational terms, linking ethical responsibility to intergenerational stewardship, community reciprocity, and cosmic balance. These are not easily quantifiable into statistical measures but they form part of every narrative of justice that pretends to be international. In the case of contemporary environmental indicators, as may be seen, sustainability is frequently measured in carbon credits or efficiency of resources, two standards that are still anchored in economistic thinking. These actions exclude the moral and spiritual aspect of the land and nature that is core to indigenous law. While initiatives like New Zealand's Living Standards Framework or Canada's First Nations Well-Being Index represent attempts to integrate indigenous perspectives into national indicator systems, however, without shared epistemic authority, without the power to define the categories themselves, these efforts risk remaining tokenistic. It is structural inclusion and not cosmetic diversity that should be the point of departure in reimagining global indicators.

Feminist and decolonial critiques make this challenge more profound by revealing how even the supposedly neutral indicators tend to reassert the epistemic and material hierarchies of the colonial modernity. María Lugones' (2010) notion of the "coloniality of gender" highlights how Western binaries, abstract individualism, and patriarchal norms distort the realities of colonized women. Measurement-wise, this implies that the relational subjectivities and embodied forms of knowledge organizing many non-Western lifeworlds cannot be measured when indicators are created around the universal male subject, the atomized nuclear household, or the economized self. Feminist interventions insist on metrics that recognize unpaid labor, community caregiving, and collective well-being—domains systematically undervalued in capitalist and development-oriented frameworks (Federici, 2020). This reorientation must involve an epistemic and institutional transformation: justice indicators must be answerable not to remote technocratic institutions, but directly to grassroots actors rooted in the daily conflicts of the communities they are claimed to represent.

The issue of responsibility invokes the global system of indicators that has continued to be influenced by institutions like United Nations, the OECD and the World Bank. While these bodies present themselves as neutral arbiters of global development and justice, critics (like Pogge) (2002) have shown how their normative frameworks and economic policies frequently entrench the very inequalities they purport to address. This dynamism suggests the necessity of what could be called metric sovereignty: the ability of communities and nations to develop, modify, or even refuse worldwide measures of indicators in light of local epistemic and normative systems. The sovereignty of metrics does not imply epistemic relativism, i.e., that any claim to justice is subject to criticism, but instead deliberative pluralism, i.e., that plural traditions can engage together in dialogue and translation and be accountable to one another. This sovereignty would create far-reaching changes in governing global justice. It is possible rather than a vertical system where there is imposition of metrics, it is possible that such a horizontal network of epistemic exchange exists where there is a co-construction of indicators through maintained dialogue across cultures, across languages, histories. This would imply that justice will not only be gauged upon communities but also be defined along with communities; in processes as pluralistic as they are politically inclusive. Globally distributed justice indicators, in whatever form, in this model are no longer instruments of homogenization, they are instruments of intercultural translation in the sense that they prevent rather than eliminate difference.

The problem of producing post-Western indicators of global justice is thus not purely technical, but profoundly philosophical. It involves giving up the myth that there exists one common measure that can entrap the moral nuance of justice by cutting across cultures and time. In its place, it demands a reflexive, dialogical model of measurement, grounded in epistemic humility, dedicated to cognitive justice, and able to acknowledge the pluriverse as a political and moral-ethical venture. It is only by doing this that measures of global justice can avoid doubling up on what seems to be an epistemic hegemony of the present, and instead act as a portal to a possible future where measurement becomes a crossing over point between multiple worlds, instead of an obstruction to them.

Integrative Justice Metrics: Transversality Across Sectors

The modern justice indicators are all too frequently programmed and implemented in sectoral silos: health education environment, employment, all with their policies, mandates, their measurement logics, and their institutional players. This system of segregation is an architecture of convenience to the Administration and not of moral conformity. It does not reflect the reality that the flourishing of human beings depends so entirely upon each other and that displacement and disadvantage are systemic. According to Nancy Fraser (2008), distributive justice cannot be meaningfully pursued without accounting for its entanglements with recognition and participation, dimensions that frequently cut across and, indeed, spill beyond, the boundaries of traditional policy domains.

A transversal method to justice indicators, basing itself in ethical integration, systemic sensitivity, and epistemic plurality, aims at shedding light on the relational issue of injustice as well as applying an opening to further coherent, more inclusive, and morally grounded public argumentation. By transversality in this context, I mean both an intellectual and practical inclination to think of justice as a system of mutually constitutive elements, not as a group of distinct jurisdictions.

On the normative grounds, the integration argument has a non-reductionist account to its ontology of justice. Justice is not the simple sum of discrete goods but a dense interconnection of capabilities, opportunities, and relational conditions (Nussbaum, 2011; Sen, 2009). Indicators of harm in fragmented form run the risk of misdiagnosing the occurrence of harm by disassociating it with the places where it is produced and reproduced. For instance, gender injustice cannot be reduced to wage inequality (economic), underrepresentation in leadership (political), or restricted access to reproductive care (health). It is a synergistic network of depreciation and marginalization that runs concurrently on all these planes, and facilitates the other. Moral reality of injustice is therefore intersectional and mutually constitutive and a metric system that cannot record such interdependencies will be subject to a distorted vision of the social world.

This interdependency is foundational to the Capability Approach, especially as articulated by Nussbaum (2011). In this case, central capabilities, e.g., bodily health, education (including political voice), emotional integrity, control over one environment, are not parallel goods, but mutually reinforcing circumstances. The shortage in one can undermine the achievement of the other and the bolstering of some enhances the achievement of the others. This makes the Capability Approach a philosophical justification of the need to abandon siloed indicators and, instead, pursue bundled justice measure in which fields are assessed on a relative basis.

The Oxford Poverty and Human Development Initiative (OPHI) has attempted such integration through the Multidimensional Poverty Index (MPI), which combines indicators across health, education, and standard of living. This represents a methodological advance over single-dimensional poverty lines, but as Robeyns (2017) notes, the MPI still fixes weightings across contexts and underplays harms grounded in recognition and relational injustice. In this way, an ethically sufficient transversal metric would have to go beyond aggregation and toward normatively appropriate combinations, with the selection of domains, their relationships, and comparative weighting being rooted in participatory and pluralistic considerations.

The intersectoral integration is also the reaction to the situation of inequality, as all too frequently it erupts most devastatingly at the points of convergence of various deprivation. These compound injustices are not merely additive but synergistic. Biological, educational, and food insecurity create a vicious cycle of deprivation whereby ill health degrades learning, environmental risks heighten morbidity, and absence of school opportunities limit economic opportunity among underprivileged children born in a polluted urban slum. Each of the harms may be captured by standard indicators; however, without a relational framework, individual indicators fail to measure how these harms compound each other and reinforce them. Public health scholarship has developed syndemic models to explain how social, ecological, and biological factors interact to amplify disease burdens (Singer, 2009). This logic can be used as justice-oriented indicator system, to track the received impact in terms of the interaction of environmental degradation with economic deprivation and social exclusion that reinforces the structural injustices. Such a vantage point shifts the meaning of integration, which is a statistical convenience, to a moral requirement, to attempt to depict injustice as experienced and reproduced.

Yet integration brings both methodological and ethical challenges. Technically, the aggregation or interconnection between indicators poses a threat to misrepresentation as a result of the collapsing of domains without levels of conceptual sensitivity. Ethically speaking, the process of prioritizing between overlapping harms tends to resemble the imposition of one normative set of priorities that are likely to exclude culturally specific perceptions of the most important things.

Robeyns (2017) offers one pathway forward: maintain open-ended lists of capabilities or justice domains and allow weighting to be determined contextually, through democratic deliberation. This strategy does not only take heed of moral and cultural diversity but also holds integration responsible to the lives that are under assessment. Participatory processes, consistent with Sen's (2009) emphasis on public reasoning and Fraser's (2008) insistence on participatory parity, allow affected communities to articulate how domains intersect in their lived experience and how those intersections should inform indicator design. The moral obligation would be not to destroy the moral grain of any field during the creation of significant systemic relationships. Integration should not imply the obliteration into one undifferentiated ranking of distinctive injustices; but should imply mutual illumination the way education is conditioned by health, environmental justice with racial justice, and political participation with financial security.

Moreover, a transversal framework also carries implications for governance. As integrated justice indicators, there should be institutional frameworks with interconnected spans that would span sectors, and which, at this point, create walls separating policies and consequent inability to implement coordinated responses. The problem here is not merely its data interoperability, but its epistemic reorientation: policy-makers and analysts have to be trained to recognize justice issues as informational, as opposed to the allure of more narrowly defined mandates. In its absence, even the most integrated metrics are at risk of being re-assimilated by the bureaucracies divided into little pieces. Lastly, integrative justice measures should be conscious of the normative commitments of the measures themselves. Such a decision as to connect, e.g., environmental and public health consequences, is not a neutral decision nonethically, but rather represents a general picture of justice, viewing ecological and human well-being as mutually connected. The explicitness of these commitments has the advantages of not only increasing the transparency but also opening up democratic discourse on whether such linkages deserve to capture the values of the people they are attempting to measure.

Overall, the transition to integrative justice measures and away from the sector silos is not only theoretically sound but also a matter of urgency. Justice is a transversal lived thing, at the interface of economic, political, cultural, and ecological conditions. Such a measurement would necessitate relational, participatory, plural, and reflexive measurement. Such a strategy would do more than just provide a truer picture of injustice; it would also achieve the sort of cross-sector solidarity and systemic thinking that create the possibility of far-reaching change. Transversal indicators have the potential to redirect the policy to stop reactive solutions and organize strategic action that will target the structural mechanisms of disadvantage rather than count it as an audit of harm with transformative potential.

Institutional Ethics and Democratic Accountability

Governmental, judicial, or administrative institutions are not just the mere passive vehicles of Justice. They are norm-constituting agents whose design, procedures, and epistemic orientations constitute those very moral terrain upon which justice is imagined, pursued, and disputed. As Iris Marion Young (2000) has argued, institutions must be evaluated not only by their distributive outputs but also by their structural orientations: whether they empower or marginalize, include or exclude, recognize or erase. The institutional practice of justice measures is therefore not an application-neutral tool on the policy of analysis, but an ethical governance technology. Their validity lies in the ways they are made possible, in the voices that they serve, to whom and what kind of moral responsibilities they represent. Each indicator is, by implication, a statement about what qualifies as justice and how it is to be known. How indicators will be thought of and used may strengthen democratic legitimacy or consolidate epistemic domination.

Epistemic injustice is one of the most severe ethical threats to the institutional indicator design. It is the systematic underrepresentation of some groups in the definition, construction, or interpretation of justice metrics. As Miranda Fricker (2007) explains, epistemic injustice is twofold. Hermeneutical injustice is the experience of lack of adequate conceptual resources in dominant discourse to describe certain social experiences, usually the experiences of marginalized or racialized groups, thereby making them invisible through official measures. Testimonial injustice is the question of some voices being systematically discounted or refused epistemic authority. Lacking authentic participatory processes in the development of indicators, indicators can serve to legitimize elitist epistemologies at the same time disguising structural violence. The information that is not there frequently can be as ethically revealing as what is there in such a case. Amartya Sen (2009) emphasizes "public reasoning" as a central dimension of justice, arguing that legitimacy is not secured through technical rigor alone but through deliberative validation. Indicators need therefore to be co-constructed in a manner that renders them accountable to the communities they purport to serve.

Three interdependent conditions have to be satisfied so that a measure could be democratically legitimate. First, transparency: the value assumptions, normative priorities, and conceptual exclusions inherent in the design of an indicator need to be spelled out. Second, reflexivity: instruments of reflexivity should integrate reviewing and revising of evidence on a periodic basis in the face of emerging evidence, new moral perceptions, and voices of individuals who are the most affected. Third, inclusion: communities that have been silenced in history or structurally marginalized must have a substantial role in how the very measurements that they will be governed by are developed. Failure to have such conditions, the indicators of justice can easily become weapons of technocratic dominance and not of democratic empowerment. The probability of the moral legitimacy of justice measures is closely tied to the institutional design, deployment, and interpretation, and is not independent of the moral legitimacy of the institution responsible for these processes. This legitimacy cannot be reduced to procedural fairness or legal validity and have to be considered in terms of more fundamental justice-sensitive conditions: dignity, agency, representation, and redress. Nancy Fraser's (2008) three-dimensional model of justice; redistribution, recognition, and representation, offers a robust framework here. Indicators should be evaluated not only on their potential to ensure equitable allocation of resources but also on their potential to recognize heterogeneous lifeworlds and enable political voice and agency. In this viewpoint, the institution's measures should also be accountable to the surroundings in a way that the institution's decisions and implementers of the indicators are directly accountable to the people who are being measured. They must include moral vetoing powers, so that the affected communities can overturn, modify, or disregard indicators that distort their lives or continue to cause harms. They must further incorporate feedback mechanisms to the general population whereby measures will be transformed to dynamic tools of civic engagement in lieu of fixed tools of management.

However, even benevolent indicators can succumb to the danger of institutional capture where the performance management, expediency, or managerial requirements of bureaucratic efficiency warp the ethical intent of measurement. Christopher Hood (1991) warns against "metric fetishism," the tendency to equate organizational success with favorable scores on select indicators, regardless of whether those scores reflect substantive justice. Indicators can encourage superficial compliance instead of transformational change when the institutions themselves are not interested in measuring their performance but fixing the issues underlying their own performance that are moral and structural. This dynamic is reflected in the case of standardized testing in education. Systems driven by narrow performance indicators may see rising test scores while simultaneously deepening inequalities in critical thinking, cultural inclusivity, or emotional well-being (Noddings, 2003). In this case, it is not an indicator of a claim to justice but an institutional justification proxy, which is considered an administrative legible text and not one that is ethically sufficient. Preventing such capture requires epistemic vigilance and institutional humility. Indicators are not to be viewed as mechanical statements of what is just, but as temporary and democratic morals to be questioned constantly in the light of enduring ethical considerations. This demands reflexive governance: an ability of institutions not merely to apply justice indicators to assess real others, but to expose themselves to indicator-based assessment on the basis of moral standards (Land & Michalos, 2018). In addition, institutions should avoid the technocratic inclination to wall off justice indicators in bureaucratic ongoing concerns. The justice metric that is constructed and interpreted by technical experts rather than wider democratic engagement could never be morally appropriate. As opposed to that, metrics need to be democratized, decolonized, and accessible to criticism, which can be based on a variety of epistemic positions. These can include co-governance agreements with civil society, autonomous audit commissions based on community authority, and assemblies of deliberation to assess and adjust indicators based on values under dispute and manifest injustices. Institutional use of indicators thus comes in doubly with an ethical burden. First, measuring institutions have to design and implement their measures to include and empower those who should be rightfully marginalized instead of the injustices that measurement seeks to eliminate reproduced through it. Second, they have to develop a culture of accountability internally, where metrics will be perceived as invitation to the moral reflection, not closure mechanisms.

The assumption in this vision is that such justice metrics are not final verdicts handed down but discursive boundaries: points of access to shared reasoning about the ethical contours of our institutions and the societies they support. They may become essential in ensuring congruence between governance and justice, though this is only when they are incorporated in the institutions with transparency, reflexivity, inclusion, and ability to be morally responsive. In the end, an ethical question is not whether an institution employs justice indicators, it is whether those indicators are aligned with, and do further justice as a normative horizon and lived social practice. Justice measures, when conceived and managed effectively, can also bring light to inequalities, facilitate community action, and enlist institutions to their public promises. When devised incorrectly, they can instead become a tool of legitimization to systems of exclusion and domination. The intersection of institutional ethics and democratic accountability can thus boil down to one requirement: to regard justice indicators as the living moral building blocks of governance, subject to being reviewed, challenged, and co-constructed. It is only on this condition that they will serve not as bureaucratic artifacts but as agents of the ongoing democratic task of holding our institutions accountable to the requirements of justice.

Integrative Justice Metrics: Transversality Across Sectors

The design of the modern policy evaluation tends to be sectorally disaggregated, viewing health, education, environment, labor, and social inclusion as separate spheres of activity with different indicators and institutional requirements. On the one hand, such fragmentation can be convenient during administration; however, it hinders to see the systemic dependencies of injustice hide and prevents the development of integrative interventions. When conceptualized properly, justice is not limited to any area alone; it is cross-sectoral and cross-subjective and requires measures that measure the relational complexities involved in human prosperity. In that regard, the trend of nearing transversal justice metrics can be defined as a necessary step of both, an epistemological and ethical nature. The purpose of these composite indicators is to show how the concepts of deprivation, recognition, capability, and dignity are co-constitutive of each other in different policy areas. The technical difficulty is not just technical, it is fundamentally philosophical: how to quantify injustice in a way that does not flatten out moral complexity or ontological interdependence and institutional coherence.

The transversality in the measurement of justice has its most persuasive theoretical convincingness in relational ontologies that eradicate the liberal attempt of the individual subject. Emmanuel Levinas and Virginia Held argue that the human self is always already constituted through relationships of responsibility, vulnerability, and care (Levinas, 2011; Held, 2006). According to this, the disintegration of interdependence is not only a harm additional to others, such as health, education, or labor injustice but moral fabric tear. The ethics of care expressed by Held questions the atomism of prevailing paradigms of justice, by invoking the need to place the focus on measuring relational needs alongside transactional rights. This face of the Other as emphasized by Levinas imparts a moral demand that is not dependent on institutional distribution—a demand of signs that makes visible, not concealed, human vulnerability and interrelatedness. The metrics required are those that are sensitive to cross-domain harms and systems-level disempowerment that are not just cumulative losses, but broken moral actions, which need integrative restoration.

Empirical observation points out the need of such integration with the finding being that injustice within one domain often leads to disadvantage in other places. Poor educational attainment correlates strongly with diminished health outcomes (Marmot, 2015); environmental degradation disproportionately affects laborers in extractive industries (Schlosberg, 2007); and structural unemployment contributes both to psychosocial distress and to reduced political agency (Sen, 1999). However, these interdependencies are not ethically sound, andare thus reflected in the limited structured data available. Composite indices such as the Human Development Index or the Multidimensional Poverty Index partially integrate multiple deprivations, but they often rely on fixed weightings or treat domains as commensurable silos (Robeyns, 2017). What a really integrative justice measure would do would be to get past aggregation and into a relationally effective encoding of intersectoral interactions. In another example, one can imagine a Relational Capability Score that measures the skills that individuals have to access education as a measure of their environmental security, or to engage in labor as a measure of their mental health and status within the polity. Similarly, a Justice Ecosystem Indicator could include but not be restricted to inputs, including resources, or outputs, including attainment and at the same time include relational conditions as trust, voice, dignity, and collective agency across the life domains.

The philosophical change is as drastic as the methodological one that is necessitated by transversality. The dominant mode of indicator design aggregates standardized data into composite scores, but aggregation often obscures intersectional harms and produces what Sally Engle Merry (2011) calls the "flattening effect" of numeric abstraction. Relational mapping and transversal strategies promote an alternative methodology of feedback loops, causal entangles, mutually reinforcing deprivation, however. This kind of approach might borrow aspects of systems theory, network analysis, and participatory mapping to enable justice indicators to map the moral geography of disadvantage. Of equal importance, by offering the advantage of relating injustice not as a series of isolated failures but as interrelated losses in human thriving, a more morally textured quantitative scale is reinstated to the quantitative scale with which the problem of injustice is nowadays gauged, generating a more truthful representation of how injustice develop and endure.

Realizing this approach also requires significant institutional redesign. Different governance structures are usually cumulatively siloed as we have ministries of health, education, environment, and labor, having their own budget, indicators, and accountability regimes. Justice metrics that span domains must be accompanied by interministerial coordination, shared epistemic platforms, and cross-sectoral deliberative mechanisms that make it possible to address harms whose origins and impacts cut across institutional boundaries (Fraser, 2008). Also, responsibility has to be a shared one: when injustice is created by the convergence of sectors then remedy must be created by the same. This necessitates governance frameworks where transversal justice indicators give rise to mutual moral commitment among the institutional actors and overcome the bureaucratic nature of passing blame among silos.

The normative reason to think integrative metrics as opposed to siloed metrics is because they disclose what siloed measures cannot, namely, that justice is not a modular accomplishment, but a moral whole. Amartya Sen (2009) observes that a just society is not one that maximizes scores on any single measure but one that sustains the conditions for public reasoning, plural valuation, and shared human flourishing. Relational indicators maintain this vision because they reveal the moral ecology of justice: how the vulnerability in one field, environmental insecurity, in this case, can have knock-ons elsewhere, undermining dignity, participation, and agency. Through plotting these interdependencies, transversal metrics render visible the incredible architecture of harm, and enable us to diagnose the loci of intervention, which can result in systemic rather than partial change. The twenty-first-century quest to seek justice demands the relinquishment of the comfort of the metrics that divide the world into logistically manageable pieces. It demands adopting a relational paradigm according to which an indicator should become characterized by the position of moral infrastructures, as scaffoldings of recognition, redistribution, and representation, of all areas of life. They are not technical devices but normative pronouncements on who counts, what matters, and how the fabric of social life ethically should be woven. The validity of their statistical accuracy is just one aspect, but this is sufficient to permit them to pay their respect to human interdependence with equivalence of moral probity.

In this vein, integrative justice measures should be interpreted as epistemic as well as ethical novelties. Epistemically, they subvert the cognitive habits of fragmentation that predominate in policy analysis. Ethically they give us a vision of justice where harms cannot be counted, as they are only pieces in a connected pattern of social, political, and environmental circumstances. They also allow us to broaden our understandings of injustice and how to respond to it, since such metrics can shape actual responses to it as well as our perceptions thereof. It is a challenging job, but the payoff is clearer, more inclusive, and ethically sound approach to justice, the approach which does not divide human flourishing into separate policy compartments and quantifies human flourishing as relational whole that it is.

Participatory Indicator Frameworks: Institutionalizing Democratic Epistemologies

The Justice measurement process is never a purely technical or administrative exercise; it is eminently epistemological and normative. As Nancy Fraser (2008) reminds us, the legitimacy of justice claims depends not only on the distribution of resources or recognition of identities, but also on who participates in defining the terms of evaluation. This emphasis aligns closely with Miranda Fricker's (2007) account of epistemic justice, which highlights the moral obligation to acknowledge and incorporate marginalized knowledge perspectives into the processes through which understanding and judgment are formed. It is in this sense that metric co-construction of justice is not just a question of consultation but of philosophical mandate to justify democratic authority. Those indicators that are created without the involvement of those they purport to represent have a potential to reproduce epistemic power gaps, strengthen social stratifications, and limit the moral domain of what ought to be considered just.

Historically, traditional metric systems objectify people and communities by viewing them as a subject of measure, what can be measured, surveyed, classified, and quantified. The epistemic architecture assumes that it will be arranged in a hierarchy where only experts will dictate what is counted, how it will be counted, and why it is important. With such a model, the hermeneutical marginalization, judging some parts of the world as having insufficient interpretive resources applied to them, is reproduced, and there is a risk of what can be called epistemic extractivism, the harvesting of data on communities without having to give them interpretive power or political voice. A move toward participatory indicators framework entails reconstituting such measurement objects of subjects of measurement as co-producers of meaning.

Deliberative platforms such as citizen assemblies, deliberative mini-publics (Fung, 2003), and community-based participatory research offer methodological pathways toward such epistemic inclusion. Such methods encourage togetherness in norm articulation so that affected communities can decide on which areas of justice are most important and how the manifestation of justice should be measured in metric binaries (Maurya, 2025). Community involvement in this case does not carry a figurative meaning; it amounts to the epistemic-moral legitimacy of the indicators themselves. By engaging citizens in defining the objects, dimensions, and purposes of measurement, not only do the citizens exert their characteristic influence on the results but they also assist in shaping the moral ontology of justice, which the metrics is supposed to reflect.

Institutional design innovations that go beyond piecemeal consultation would be needed to turn democratic epistemologies into practice at the indicator level. The process of creating measurement should incorporate deliberative infrastructure via open, inclusive spaces where dissimilar groups of persons can discuss long-term dialogues regarding the values and priorities of the measurement. This sort of infrastructuring would imply interpretive accessibility, by using linguistic and cultural diversity, hermeneutical equity, translating technical language, and enhancing contextual education. Rotating knowledge panels can institutionalize a diversity of perspectives, ensuring that indigenous, feminist, disabled, working-class, and other marginalized lifeworlds are represented in metric design. These panels are capable of avoiding epistemic closure by cyclically changing membership, refreshing an ever-new infusion of plural views.

Equally important are mechanisms for auditability and contestability. The metrics should not be given the primacy of being factual but as tentative and subject to further revision in the eyes of the public. Institutions should have channels of formal critique, grievance, and revision, and indicators should be living tools called upon to act according to changing realities moral and political. This resonates with Boaventura de Sousa Santos's (2014) call for cognitive justice, not only the recognition of multiple epistemologies but also the creation of institutional scaffolding capable of sustaining them in practice.

Participatory indicator frameworks also serve an educative role. By inviting citizens into the act of defining justice, they operate as civic pedagogies, cultivating deliberative capacities, enhancing public reasoning (Sen, 2009), and developing a shared language of justice. In a pluralistic society, such participatory processes are required in particular where justice claims are articulated on the basis of opposing cosmologies, historical traumas, and vocabularies of morality. Against this background, indicator co-construction turns into an act of democratic mediation, where the negotiation of competing visions can occur without epistemic violence. The educative dimension extends further into the development of what Paulo Freire (1970) called critical consciousness, the capacity to interrogate structures of power, resist technocratic domination, and reclaim agency in shaping policy. Participatory metrics not only democratize knowledge production, in this sense, but also develop civic capacities of participating in the production of knowledge, that is, all required to maintain democratic life itself.

The possibilities to integrate participation in the design of metrics have been illustrated with several modern programs. The Wellbeing Economy Alliance (WEAll) and New Zealand's Wellbeing Budget, for example, have sought to engage citizens in determining the metrics by which societal progress is judged, moving beyond GDP to more holistic measures of well-being. Brazilian and Indian participatory budgeting programs give the community a place in fiscal decision-making, and provide a preview of how deliberation can inform values as well as tangible policy products. Equally, the Community-Driven Data efforts help funded by the UNDP enable marginalized populations to develop their own measures of justice, dignity, and well-being so that the act of measurement has local priorities and logics at heart.

These examples indicate that democratic renewal can be a factor at the stage of metric construction and not necessarily as a point of bureaucratic perfection. Indicators can be turned into a means of empowering citizens and not watching them or controlling them when they are not only active in the provision of data, but in the definition of what the data means. Participatory structures in this way displace the epistemic center of gravity and redistribute the power to determine how justice is to be defined, measured, and sought. The normative argument on participatory indicators systems is more than legitimacy to morality. These frameworks represent a theory of justice in which knowledge is considered to be relational, lived experiences are thought to be irreductible, and all epistemic agents have dignity in their existence. They discredit the instrumental rationality of measurement as limited managerial tools and recover the objectification of managerial devices as moral-political practices based on dialogue and mutual detection. Through this, they index the measurement to the ethical necessities of inclusion, respect, and co-ownership of the common good.

The practice of designing indicators thus needs to be reconceptualized as not a technically neutral activity but an ethically dense one. Participatory frameworks provide one route to achieving justice-sensitive epistemologies because they serve to put political and moral stakes at the center of indicator-making. Measurement can only be regarded as just when it captures the voice and values of those that experience their consequences. In democracy institutionalizing democratic epistemologies, we not only democratize the process that administers the ongoing project of measurement, but we universalize the exigence of historical justice itself as a lived, contested, and collaboratively authored venture.

The Role of Technology and AI in Justice Metrics

The integration of Artificial Intelligence (AI) and algorithmic systems into justice-oriented governance marks a turning point in moral epistemology. Whether about crime hotspots, educational inequity extremities, or health disparities modeling, AI-enabled indicators are becoming key to how institutions spend dollars and how improvement is measured. Though such systems are envisaged to be efficient, scalable, and adaptive in decision-making, they also require ruminative philosophical examination. Algorithms can never be neutral; they reflect normative assumptions and assigns different values and define our image of justice as such. Their addition to justice metrics is not an incidental technical enrichment of justice, but an extreme revision of moral responsibility.

Algorithmic indicators scale extremely large datasets to determine trends and to produce predictive analytics in all domains, including housing, policing, education, and health care. By pointing out trends of injustice that elude other means of traditional discernment, such predictive power comes to indicate avenues of great epistemological danger. Arcane historical biases that are present in the data are usually mathematically re-encoded into algorithmic outputs. As Cathy O'Neil (2016) and Ruha Benjamin (2019) have shown, machine learning models trained on biased data reproduce and even amplify inequities. A widely cited example is the COMPAS risk assessment tool in the US criminal justice system, which predicted higher recidivism risk for Black defendants than for white defendants with similar profiles. Under those circumstances, technological systems are naturalized types of structural racism, with claims to be the purification of empirical objectivity. This provokes a refutation of the popular idea that the metrics of justice can be developed without reflexivity and historical consciousness (Maurya, 2024). Many AI systems are "black boxes" whose internal decision-making logic is inaccessible even to their designers (Burrell, 2015). This unintelligibility misplaces responsibility and causes a case where, when decisions that are of a normative significance are made, due to the fact that the decision was made by a non-sentient system then, in a real sense, the moral decision is taken out of human hands. Normatively, this brings the issue of moral delegation; is normative judgment possible to be held by an algorithm? According to Mark Coeckelbergh, the responsibility belongs to moral agents, not computational tools, and that outsourcing moral reasoning to machines risks eroding the accountability structures that underpin justice (Coeckelbergh, 2020). Nonetheless, despite such risks, AI can lead toward enhanced justice measures when incorporated into ethical responsible governance. A potential usage can be made in the improvement of deliberative foresight by means of scenario-based simulations. The long-term distributive impacts of alternative policy decisions and machine learning can provide predictive information on the impacts of policy interventions on different groups of people. For example, predictive justice simulations can reveal how environmental regulations may have unintended impacts on marginalized labor sectors, enabling more anticipatory and inclusive policy-making (Guston, 2014). Such tools can function as "moral imagination by proxy" (Miller, 2019), helping decision-makers explore the ethical implications of policy options before they are enacted.

Nevertheless, AI should always be an epistemic scaffold instead of becoming a moral legislator. Moral judgment in the Kantian tradition must be autonomous, self-reflective, and norm-responsive, traits that machines lack. Elizabeth Anderson (1993) argues that ethical judgment is grounded in empathic perspective-taking, something no algorithm, however complex, can authentically simulate. Moreover, justice is not reducible to computational outputs; it is a social practice embedded in historical memory, narrative, and recognition (Honneth, 1996). Machines are not in a position to have lived experience to recognize moral injuries, symbolic harms, or offenses to dignity, which are one of the focuses of recognition-based theories of justice.

This philosophical boundary underscores the importance of Value-Sensitive Design (Friedman et al., 2002), a framework for integrating moral and political values into technological development. Within the field of metrics of justice, Value-Sensitive Design requires sharing the AI system through co-creation with the various and impacted stakeholders and should see the assumptions guiding the AI aligned with plural epistemologies of justice. Virginia Dignum (2019) extends this into the realm of Responsible AI, emphasizing transparency, accountability, inclusiveness, and contextual fairness. More practically, it can be translated into algorithms that can be understood by both engineers and the people whose lives it is accounting; audit tools against the unfair results; ethical pluralist that would not allow entrenching a single, hegemonic sense of justice. These principles align with Joshua Cohen's (1989) vision of deliberative democracy, where legitimacy arises from inclusive public reasoning rather than technocratic fiat.

In the absence of such protections, the dangers of AI do not lie in ostensible technocratic rule; rather they are in the form of new entrenched normative biases, which have the effect of closing off contestation. It can become useful in working with them to map inequities, to model policy effects, and to maintain a participatory politics of measurement. The complexity is not whether or not to use AI as a measure of justice, but on what normative terms it will be running and what about its governance? How can the human moral agency not be subordinate to AI?

Ultimately, AI and algorithmic indicators are conditional technologies within overall moral ecologies. Their moral authority has less to do with technical savvy than with conformity with human dignity, agency, and deliberative responsibility. It is interesting to note that the idea of justice is not something that can be automated and be a machine product; rather it is a human accomplishment with the use of information, never machine-dictated. However, the online transition in the measuring of justice is a chance and a warning. AI, properly designed, can serve to show the systemic injustice and open up the vista of moral imagination. It is ill-managed and poses danger of establishing inequity itself. The critical question is: are we in the process to adopt these tools still faithful to democratic and philosophical roots of justice itself?

Philosophical Reorientation: Beyond Perfectionism, Toward a Critical Utopianism

The cultures of policy and epistemic around justice metrics might be dominated by perfectionist assumptions, in other words that justice constitutes a final state whose degree can be attained by designing the institution of justice appropriately and measured by optimal indicators. Those organizations are reminiscent of the teleological moral theories, which envision justice as a steady state, something that can be achieved, measured against, and maintained after its acquisition. Although it is administratively desirable, this model is very philosophically limiting as well as misleading. As Jacques Derrida reminds us in *Force of Law* (1993), justice is "that which is to come," a promise that resists closure, totalization, or full articulation. In contrast to law that can be codified and applied, justice is open, an endless horizon to which ethically it is impertinent that we have access. Efforts to fix, conclude, or capture justice in any given set of indicators threaten the closure of metaphysics that, according to Derrida, denies (the other) alterity by obliterating futurity (Maurya, 2022). This observation demands the hermeneutic suspicion of claims of the possibility of measuring justice on a conclusive basis. Indictors are not expected to achieve reified status as the epochal account of the true moral accomplishment; but should serve as placeholders in the struggle, as staging posts in the process of cultural amelioration.

By adopting a becoming rather than completion view of justice we do not turn our back on normativity. On the contrary, it deepens moral responsibility. This orientation resonates with process philosophy (Whitehead, 1929), which views value as a dynamic unfolding rather than a fixed essence. Justice according to this register cannot be understood as a stagnant practice that is fixed or determined by history, struggles about the law, and plural ambitions. It cannot be rigorously crystallized into any one assessment structure without jeopardizing the preclusion of voices, harms, or avenues that may be realized with time.

Nancy Fraser (2008) advances a similar point: justice claims are historically situated and must remain open to revision in light of new exclusions or injustices. In this light, indicators are only temporary, debatable, normative assumptions instead of fixed judgments. They are always answerable to future critique. This type of attitude undermines technocratic trust in the right set of measurements and shifts into a reflexive style: any measurement is precarious and can be reinstated. Rejecting perfectionism does not render indicators useless. Utopia, in this case, is less like a pipedream of unrealizable plans than a critical form of political imagination: a place to imagine the possibility of other worlds. This utopian role can be played by indicators, which when relieved of the burden of finality can play this indicative role. They can serve as a tool of diagnosing injustice in both emergent and systemic form, generating moral imagination of what more just world can look like, and setting a table of deliberative opportunity to visualize forms of political possibility quite different than now. They do not close debates; they provoke them. Such re-ontologization of indicators can be done without their re-ontologization as neutral measurement tools; rather, as ethico-political artifacts. The very markers of indicators also lie within the value fights, institutional preferences, and the disputed idealizations of the societies that generate them. As such, their evaluation must extend beyond statistical validity to include normative transparency (are the underlying values made explicit?), dialogical openness (do they invite dissent and reinterpretation?), and moral resonance (do they reflect the lived realities and aspirations of diverse communities?). In this sense, indicators are not the goal but the stage, the place of the negotiation between different visions of justice, which struggle to obtain legitimacy. Not only should they be evaluated on the basis of how they create all-inclusive conversation but also on their technical accuracy. Whether they provide an ideal image of justice is of course the question, but not whether they intensify shared involvement in the work of seeking it. On this critical-utopian horizon, measurement does not focus so much on closure as on orientation. Indicators do not map what justice is, but the sketches of what it might be. They are also intermediate maps to an incomplete horizon with the realization that the landscape will morph as we approach it. This requires both designers and those who use metrics to be humble indeed: to the acknowledgment that any indicator is only a slice of reality, through the lenses and valuation interests of the constructors.

The justice-to-come points out that there are temptations to treat justice as a finished thing that must be avoided. It demands that we look carefully again and again over how our existing actions potentially blind us to new forms of evil or stifle alternative imaginings. A perfectionist measure dangerously may lock justice into a specific pattern, turning justice, which must be an idea vitalized, into institutionalized bureaucratic relic (Maurya, 2021). Critical-utopian metric, in its turn, works with its own provisionality; it takes provisionality as a fuel of moral imagination and political regeneration.

The philosophic transition away from perfectionism and toward critical utopianism has on its side a reconstitution not only of the standards of justice, but their subsequent positioning within an open-ended democratic practice. Indicators turn into collective orientation projects, rather than judgments of collective arrival. Then they are not meant to answer the question of the end of moral struggle, but merely that it should be kept alive, the points are to be raised, the tensions to be aroused, the resources to be made available enabling societies to practice their own futures, which could not at the time perhaps be truly attained. After all, measuring justice is not to understand it. It is to pursue it—not as a final destination or endpoint, but as a guide, urging us toward higher aspirations. This necessitates designing and reading indicators as an invitation to conversation and not a statement of conclusiveness; as an artifact that keeps the option of surprise, resistance, and re-imagination open. Justice is never final, but always in the making. The truth must be able to translate onto our metrics or they will end up betraying the very ideal they are designed to serve.

Concluding Summary

The movement charted in this book has been philosophical as well as practicable. The transition in this book has been one between ontological and epistemological justification, of justice on the one hand and empirical assessment of the demands of justice on the other hand through metrics as well as critical-constructive forecast of an indicative stance that ought to prevail in the future. What has not arisen is any single, monolithic evaluative metric, but instead an alternative metrology of justice plural, self-defining, and reflexively appreciating its own role in the great game of measurability: A tolerant of necessity, and yet a vigorous opponent, of the peculiar reductionism to which quantification lends itself in the shared affairs of social life. In an argument presented here justice is not able to be caught in any comprehensive way (Maurya, 2020). It is neither an exhaustive collection of distributive arrangements nor is it an exhaustively achievable situation. Following Sen (2009) and Fraser (2008), justice is best understood as a meta-norm, a critical orientation that animates the design, interpretation, and contestation of indicators. In that spirit, indicators are not fixed judgments, but instead moving appeals to moral reflection, whose purpose is to offer provocation toward normative inquiry, rather than to close it. The integration of the theory and the sensitivity of the empirical hence provides a methodological posture based on deference, challengeability, and participatory plurality.

In much contemporary governance, indicators are being used as technocratic finalities, figures that identify success or failure, facilitate interjurisdictional comparison and act as the driver of accountability. However this instrumentalist stance threatens to make the deliberative aspects of the public life to disappear. It narrows the "public space of appearance" described by Arendt (1958), the arena in which individuals collectively deliberate on shared values and the common good. The vision that is promoted here is not the same: the indicators are to be perceived as the moral provocations. They should shed light on injustices that have been concealed through prevalent paradigms, reveal the voices of the marginalized communities, and disrupt comforting stories of development. These indicators are not as much a performance management instrument as they are an impetus to moral and political dialogue. They do not offer closure; they open up openings on contestation and imagination as well as collective thinking. In this broader sense, a justice measure is not a response, rather it is a moral query in figures.

The Moral Architecture of Future Indicators

To serve genuinely just futures, indicators must be grounded in a moral architecture built upon three interlocking commitments:

Dignity A just indicator affirms the irreducibility of the human person. It resists forms of abstraction that erase the context, narrative, or subjectivity of those it measures (Nussbaum, 2011). The work of measurement is not neutral, it carries moral weight, and the act of quantifying should never undermine the worth or agency of the individuals and communities under observation.

Plurality Justice is never singular. Competing philosophical traditions—libertarian, egalitarian, communitarian, feminist, decolonial—each bring partial yet indispensable insights. Indicators should be built to reflect this normative pluralism, resisting the imposition of a single hegemonic ideal. As Santos (2014) argues in his call for "epistemologies of the South," a truly just metric culture must incorporate diverse ways of knowing, multiple ontologies of well-being, and heterogeneous visions of flourishing.

Collective Responsibility Justice is not an individual virtue but a shared obligation. Indicators should be framed to emphasize interdependence, relationality, and institutional accountability. This requires embedding metric design in processes of public reasoning, co-construction, and ongoing revision, an ethics of measurement that evolves through civic participation rather than elite imposition (Sen, 2009; Fricker, 2007).

From Descriptive Statistics to Normative Imagination

The final and conclusive normative shift is simple: guides should not simply describe how the world is, they should assist us in imagining how the world ought to be. Measurement should cultivate what Taylor (2003) calls "moral horizons," background frameworks that shape our sense of what is worthy of pursuit, indignation, and repair. In this spirit, indicators become sites of utopian pedagogy (Levitas, 2013), tools that not only record conditions but also train our moral imagination, orienting political action toward a justice that is always, in Derrida's (1993) phrase, à venir, "to come." It implies avoiding the urge to judge metrics as adequate manifestation of justice. Rather, all indicators are considered to be tentative maps, never comprehensive and subject to redesign based on novel types of exclusion, recognition, and redistribution. To measure well, therefore, is not to calculate better, it is to pose better moral questions. Statistical soundness is not the only criteria to measure the validity of an indicator, which has to be ethically vibrant. No matter how accurate, a figure that drowns out complication or eliminates discord is the figure of an authority that is without recourse to morality.

From Quantification to Ethical Orientation

The central argument of this book is that indicators are not mere technical artifacts since they lack neutrality. They are moral grammars, narratives, frames, and symbol schemes to give ideas about just and the way societies imagine, seek, and judge. In order to cultivate measurable moral futures, we have to incorporate justice measures in a philosophy that ascertains dignity, plurality, and maintenance of democratic responsibility. Instead of running after the elusive ideal of the coveted silver bullet indicator, we need to develop critical, pluralistic, and participatory metric cultures, ones that leave the option of contestation and revision, ones that understand justice as a collective horizon, and not a procedural endgame. Only thus can our striving to quantify justice escape betrayal of the ideal that the striving attempts to serve. It should never be an action of moral fidelity," every action of the same is a continuing act, which is held to follow justice, not end with its completion. The thing is, after all, not to make our numbers perfect, but to find them restless and keep them honest and at work on justice, always in the making.

References

Anderson, E. (1993). *Value in ethics and economics*. Harvard University Press.

Arendt, H. (1958). *The human condition*. University of Chicago Press.

Benjamin, R. (2019). *Race after technology: Abolitionist tools for the new Jim code*. Polity.

Berlin, I. (1969). *Four essays on liberty*. Oxford University Press.

Burrell, J. (2015). How the machine "thinks": Understanding opacity in machine learning algorithms. *Big Data & Society, 3*(1).

Coeckelbergh, M. (2020). *AI ethics*. MIT Press.

Derrida, J. (1993). Force of law: The "Mystical Foundation of Authority". In D. Cornell, M. Rosenfeld, & D. Gray Carlson (Eds.), *Deconstruction and the possibility of justice*. Routledge.

Dignum, V. (2019). *Responsible artificial intelligence: How to develop and use AI in a responsible way*. Springer.

Federici, S. (2020). *Revolution at point zero: Housework, reproduction, and feminist struggle*. PM Press.

Fraser, N. (2008). *Scales of justice: Reimagining political space in a globalizing world*. Polity Press.

Friedman, B., Kahn, P., & Borning, A. (2002). *Value sensitive design: Theory and methods*. University of Washington Technical Report.

Fung, A. (2003). Recipes for public spheres: Eight institutional design choices and their consequences. *Journal of Political Philosophy, 11*(3), 338–367.

Guston, D. H. (2014). Understanding 'Anticipatory Governance'. *Social Studies of Science, 44*(2), 218–242.

Held, V. (2006). *The ethics of care: Personal, political, and global*. Oxford University Press.

Honneth, A. (1996). *The struggle for recognition: The moral grammar of social conflicts*. Polity Press.

Hood, C. (1991). A public management for all seasons? *Public Administration, 69*(1), 3–19.

Jonas, H. (1984). *The imperative of responsibility: In search of an ethics for the technological age*. University of Chicago Press.

Levinas, E. (2011). *Totality and infinity: An essay on exteriority*. Duquesne University Press.

Land, K. C., & Michalos, A. C. (2018). Fifty years after the social indicators movement: Has the promise been fulfilled? *Social Indicators Research, 135*(3), 835–868. https://doi.org/10.1007/s11205-017-1571-y

Levitas, R. (2013). *Utopia as method: The imaginary reconstitution of society*. Palgrave Macmillan.

Lugones, M. (2010). The Coloniality of gender. *Worlds & knowledges otherwise*, Spring 2010.

Marmot, M. (2015). The health gap: The challenge of an unequal world. Bloomsbury.

Maurya, S. K. (2025). Restorative justice and karmic justice: Ubuntu and Vedanta in dialogue. *African Journal of Religion, Philosophy and Culture, 6*(2).

Maurya, S. K. (2024). African philosophies of justice and equity: A contemporary discourse. *African Journal of Religion, Philosophy and Culture, 5*(2), 61–78. https://doi.org/10.31920/2634-7644/2024/v5n2a4

Maurya, S. K. (2022). On just, justice and distributive justice: A critical and comparative discourse. *Journal of Liberty and International Affairs, 8*(2), 240–254. https://doi.org/10.47305/JLIA2282240m

Maurya, S. K. (2021). The concept of justice in reference with philosophies of Plato and Aristotle: A critical study. *Journal of Liberty and International Affairs, 7*(3), 250–266. https://doi.org/10.47305/JLIA21370250m
Maurya, S. K. (2020). A reply to Louis P. Pojman's article "The case against affirmative action". *Conatus—Journal of Philosophy, 5*(2), 87–113.
Merry, S. E. (2011). Measuring the world: Indicators, human rights, and global governance. *Current Anthropology, 52*(S3), S83–S95.
Merry, S. E. (2016). *The seductions of quantification: Measuring human rights, gender violence, and sex trafficking*. University of Chicago Press.
Miller, R. (2018). *Transforming the future: Anticipation in the 21st century*. UNESCO Publishing.
Miller, T. (2019). Explanation in artificial intelligence: Insights from the social sciences. *Artificial Intelligence, 267*, 1–38.
Noddings, N. (2003). *Caring: A feminine approach to ethics and moral education*. University of California Press.
Nussbaum, M. C. (2011). *Creating capabilities: The human development approach*. Harvard University Press.
O'Neil, C. (2016). *Weapons of math destruction: How Big Data increases inequality and threatens democracy*. Crown.
Pogge, T. (2002). *World poverty and human rights*. Polity Press.
Robeyns, I. (2017). *Wellbeing, freedom and social justice: The capability approach re-examined*. Open Book Publishers.
Santos, B. d. S. (2014). *Epistemologies of the south: Justice against epistemicide*. Routledge.
Schlosberg, D. (2007). Defining environmental justice: Theories, movements, and nature. Oxford University Press.
Sen, A. (1999). *Development as freedom*. Oxford University Press.
Sen, A. (2009). *The idea of justice*. Harvard University Press.
Singer, M. (2009). *Introduction to syndemics: A critical systems approach to public and community health*. Jossey-Bass.
Taylor, C. (2003). *Modern social imaginaries*. Duke University Press.
Whyte, K. (2018). Indigenous climate change studies: Indigenizing futures, decolonizing the anthropocene. *English Language Notes, 56*(1), 153–162.
Whitehead, A. N. (1929). *Process and reality: An essay in cosmology*. Macmillan.

MIX
Papier aus verantwortungsvollen Quellen
Paper from responsible sources
FSC® C105338

If you have any concerns about our products,
you can contact us on
ProductSafety@springernature.com

In case Publisher is established outside the EU,
the EU authorized representative is:
Springer Nature Customer Service Center GmbH
Europaplatz 3, 69115 Heidelberg, Germany

Printed by Libri Plureos GmbH
in Hamburg, Germany